Shakira Akabusi is a pre- and po[st] ... r
and the founder of **StrongLikeM**[um]

Mum of four (Rio, Ezra and twins ...
passionate about sharing expert k[n]
postnatal health to empower women to build confidence and positivity
during their motherhood experience. Alongside supporting women in
maintaining a healthy lifestyle, Shakira is on a mission to shatter the
stereotypes surrounding motherhood, in particular body image and
mental wellbeing.

Qualified in pre- and postnatal exercise and certified as an advanced
postnatal practitioner, Shakira is proud of bringing together a growing
community of women through **StrongLikeMum**, and is committed to
supporting mothers to achieve their goals in sports, business, lifestyle
and all areas of parenthood.

'I wish this book was out when I was pregnant for the first time, especially for all the tips about dealing with pre-natal morning sickness and post-natal exhaustion. Shakira's cheerleading voice would have helped me understand why my body – and mind – were struggling with some of the changes motherhood brings, and given me the power and purpose to be my strongest and healthiest for my baby and, most importantly, me!'

Sarah Ivens, author of *The Zen Mama*

'Motivational and inspirational – everything you need to keep your body and mind fit and healthy throughout your pregnancy and beyond'

Stephanie Anthony, *Mother & Baby*

the strong like mum method

Awaken the power of your pre and postnatal body through **instinct, knowledge & exercise**

Shakira Akabusi

ROBINSON

ROBINSON

First published in Great Britain in 2022
by Robinson

10 9 8 7 6 5 4 3 2 1

Important note

This book is not intended as a substitute
for medical advice or treatment.

Any person with a condition requiring
medical attention should consult a
qualified medical practitioner or
suitable health specialist.

If you choose to engage in this exercise
program, you agree that you do so at
your own risk and assume all risk of
injury to yourself. The creators,
publishers and experts of this book
disclaim any liability or loss (to the full
extent they are legally able) arising out
of or in connection with the instruction,
services or exercise and advice herein.

A CIP catalogue record for this book
is available from the British Library.

ISBN 978-1-47214-658-8

Typeset in Sentinel, a typeface
designed by Jonathan Hoefler and
Tobias Frere-Jones in 2009.

Printed and bound in Great Britain by
Clays Ltd, Elcograf S.p.A

Papers used by Robinson are from
well-managed forests and other
responsible sources.

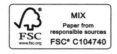

Robinson
An imprint of
Little, Brown Book Group
Carmelite House
50 Victoria Embankment
London EC4Y 0DZ
An Hachette UK Company
www.hachette.co.uk
www.littlebrown.co.uk

How To Books are published by
Robinson, an imprint of Little, Brown
Book Group. We welcome proposals
from authors who have first-hand
experience of their subjects. Please set
out the aims of your book, its target
market and its suggested contents in an
email to howto@littlebrown.co.uk

This book is undoubtedly dedicated to my children, Rio, Ezra, Aryana and Asher, and to any future children that I may have. Who continue to be the greatest teachers on how to live life with energy, passion and love in abundance.

Also for my wider family and friends, who have helped tirelessly with chapters, confidence and, most importantly, childcare so I could write this manuscript.

Finally, a part of this book is for Tracy Parkes, the midwife who helped to deliver my first son. We haven't met or spoken since that day but you guided me through the journey to becoming a mother for the first time. I hope this book can support women in a similar way to how you supported me that night.

Contents

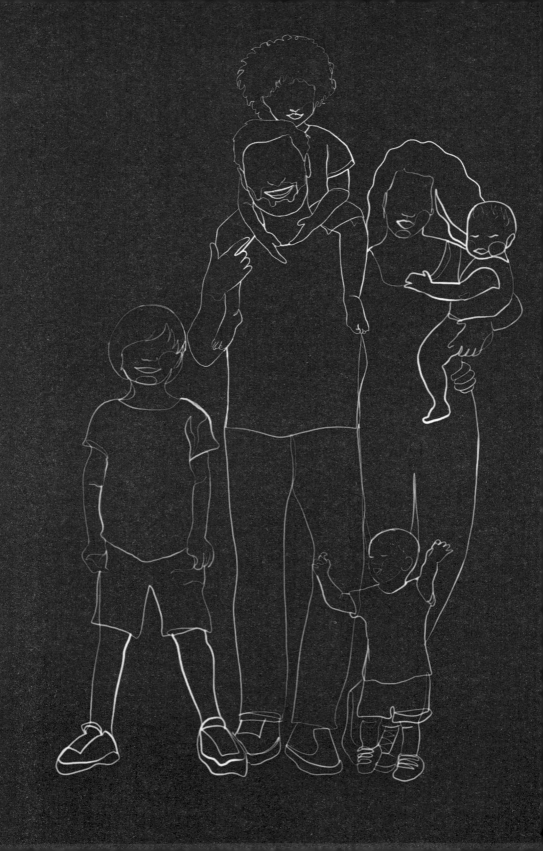

Introduction

Writing this introduction is just the strangest thing. Because it's hard to put into words how much of myself I have invested into this book. It has been part of my day-to-day life for over two years, longer if you count the very first flicker of the idea. It's been exhilarating, and at times exhausting, filling these pages with as much knowledge, experience and passion as possible. The effort is probably second only to the times I've given birth!

I first became fascinated with pregnancy, birth and motherhood about a decade ago, just before conceiving my eldest son. Since then we've added three more tiny sets of feet to our household. Over the last seven years I've experienced four pregnancies, three births, two epidurals and one caesarean section, and throughout it all I've been overwhelmingly captivated by what the female body can do. How it can create, carry, birth, heal and move. Yet, what continues to strike me is that during and after pregnancy, only minimal advice is shared about any of this.

Throughout my first pregnancy, I noticed a lack of discussion surrounding the hugely significant changes taking place in the female body during this time. Like the drastic hormonal imbalances, the connection of the jaw to the pelvic floor, or how our mental wellbeing can impact the speed of our recovery.

Being a pre- and postnatal exercise specialist, I believe that knowledge is the key to a healthy pregnancy and sustainable postnatal recovery, and for far too long the secrets of pre- and postnatal health have been kept between the experts. I want to break down that wall.

I guess I should briefly go back to how this all began. To the start of **StrongLikeMum** and how I came to be a fully qualified pre- and postnatal exercise specialist, sitting in my office, with four children causing a ruckus downstairs, writing a book to support women during this time of their lives.

The spark of StrongLikeMum

We decided we were going to try for a baby and then it started, almost instantaneously: other people's opinions. 'Are you sure you're ready?' 'You don't know how hard it is.' 'You'll never sleep again.' 'Say goodbye to your ab muscles.'

I'm sure if you're reading this during or after pregnancy, you'll have heard your own versions of such 'advice'. I put 'advice' in quotation marks because my understanding is that advice is usually asked for and constructive. These comments were neither.

In an effort to block out the negativity and live in the moment, I started blogging about my journey and it became apparent that I wasn't alone in feeling this way. Soon I had connected with hundreds and eventually thousands of women online. The specifics of the conversations would vary, but one common thread remained the same: the bubbling undertone of uncertainty about what their bodies were going through and how they might recover.

As this online community grew, so did my passion for pre- and postnatal health. I had been a personal trainer for five years already, specialising in pre- and postnatal health, and I was adamant that every woman should know the information I knew. Everyone should feel confident in their role as a mum, and never again should a woman worry about how she might recover after birth.

I combined my professional expertise in pre- and postnatal exercise with my passion for supporting maternal mental health. Thus, the spark that fuelled **StrongLikeMum** ignited.

What's in a name?

Isn't naming your child the toughest thing? I was very aware that the names I chose could stick with them for life, and that's how I felt about naming my blog too.

I wanted something that would make it clear that I believed mums are already strong. I didn't want to suggest mothers needed improving and it was important to me that it could also be something for children to look up to. Instead of saying, 'I want to be strong like superman', I would love the next generation to grow up thinking, 'I want to be strong like my mum'. I paused, finishing that thought: '**StrongLikeMum**, that sounds alright...'

Then, one afternoon during an interview, I was taken off guard by the question, 'Where can people contact you?' I blurted out '**StrongLikeMum.com**', and suddenly it was official. Well, almost. I hung up from the call and rushed to secure the domain name. Then I sat back and gave myself a few moments to enjoy what I'd created – a blank webpage with absolutely no content whatsoever, but a cracking good name at least!

What followed was years of 'research', also known as pregnancy! I was already qualified in pre- and postnatal exercise but for the next six years I swapped textbooks for trimesters and learned on the job.

Despite the challenges parenting can sometimes present, these years have been the best of my life and they have provided some of the best extra-curricular homework in terms of my career working in women's health.

I simply never would have been able to write this book without my children, because only now do I understand how motherhood presents obstacles to sustaining a regular fitness programme or healthy lifestyle that we don't encounter at other stages of our life.

I know that for pregnant women and new mums, it's not just about 'fitting in a workout', it's about finding a time where baby is happy to be left, so you can enjoy some solo exercise. I know how hard it is to find the energy after sleepless nights and I've lived the reality of needing to express before a jog, to ease the boulders that seem to have replaced your breasts post-birth.

It's these sticky bits of motherhood that hold the pages of this book together.

‘MY HOPE IS THAT THIS BOOK CAN SUPPORT WOMEN TO ACHIEVE OPTIMAL RECOVERY AND FEEL MORE ENERGISED, ACTIVE, FITTER, HAPPIER AND MORE CONFIDENT THAN EVER BEFORE.’

I'll be honest: half of this book has been written at my desk in peace and quiet, with a laptop and a mug of my favourite tea in hand. The other half, however, has been compiled in the car outside school, on my phone during night feeds, in a den, at the park, on the trampoline or wherever I can find five minutes' peace, which sometimes has included hiding in the loo!

My hope is that this book can support women to achieve optimal recovery and feel more energised, active, fitter and more confident than ever before.

Contrary to the warnings I was given about motherhood during my first pregnancy, the experience has been completely empowering. Yes, there can be challenges – I've had moments where I've felt overwhelmed and, dare I say it, incapable. But motherhood is one of those rare animalistic experiences where you can draw on strength you didn't even know was there.

This book has been written to give you a full understanding of what your body and mind are capable of during and after pregnancy.

I want to strip back the stereotypes and share with you the reality of what is happening. I hope that by sharing this information, every single woman will feel free to be happy and healthy, and form a motherhood journey that works for them. FREE. FROM. STEREOTYPES.

Funnily enough, as I finish this intro, one of my twins is waking up. So I'm afraid no fancy ending, but I suppose this isn't really the end of anything; it's just the beginning.

I hope you enjoy reading this book as much as I enjoyed writing it.

Shakira x

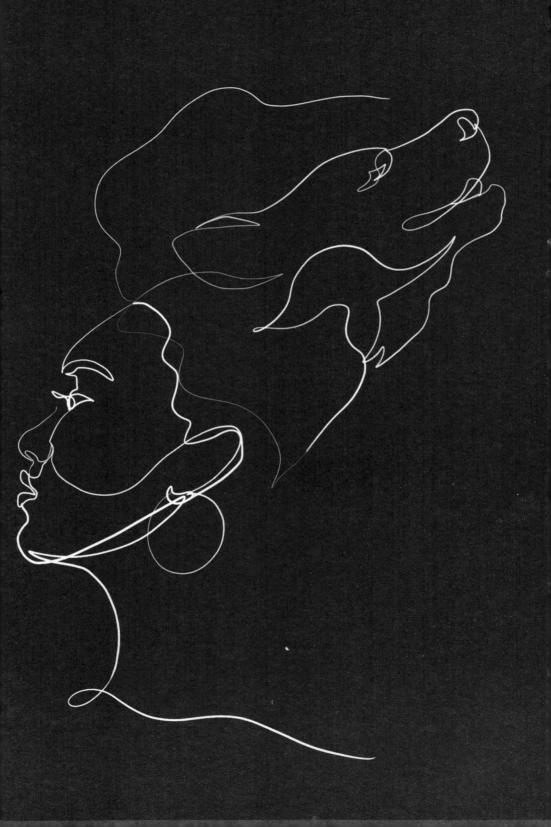

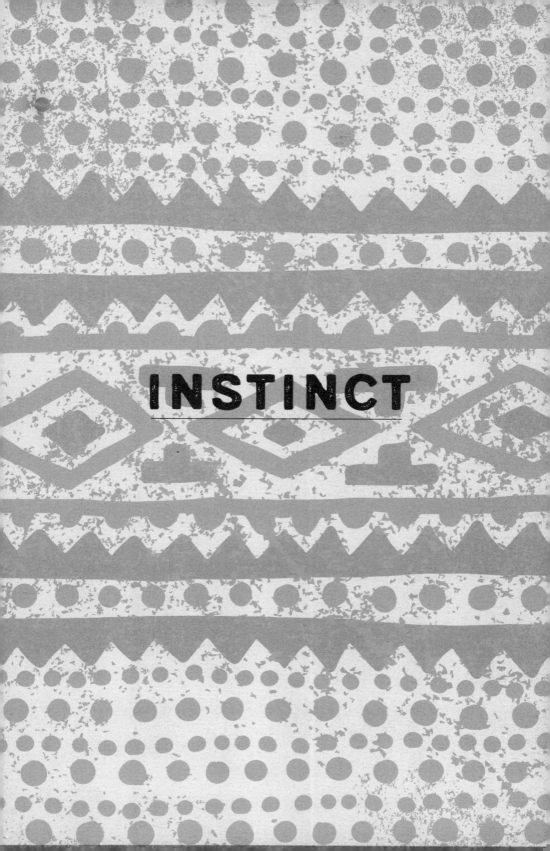

INSTINCT

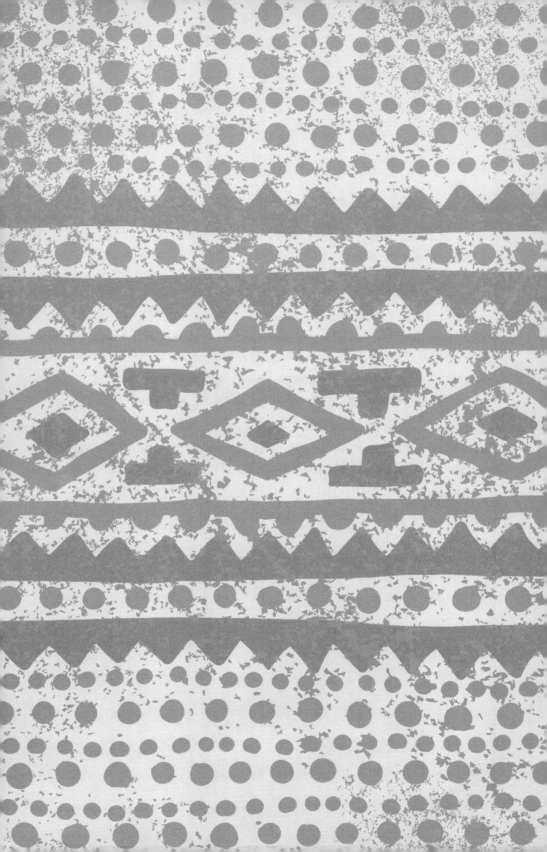

StrongLikeMum

Before words there was movement. How we move and how we feel have been aligned for millennia.

Women have also been birthing since then.

Pregnancy, birth and motherhood are undeniably a combination of both body and mind. The strength of the female frame united with the power of our psyche. The idea that our bodies are somehow weaker during pregnancy, or broken after giving birth, has never made sense to me. We've just created, carried and birthed life. Is there anything stronger?

What *is* true is that during conception, pregnancy, labour, birth and parenthood our bodies adapt in the most fascinating way. But rather than leaving us weaker, I'd argue the opposite. I believe that as mothers we can be stronger, both physically and mentally, than ever before.

The original mother

Before we can look at how our body changes during pregnancy, and what we can do to help support recovery, we need to look at how it all began. If we can understand where we've been, then we will know how best to move forwards. So, let's journey back briefly to the original mother, known as Mitochondrial Eve, aka the mother of all humans.

This might seem like a bit of a head-scratcher at first but bear with me, because it will clarify a lot about how the female body functions and why we move the way we do.

Let me start by explaining what mitochondria are, because we all have billions of them in our body. Mitochondria are teeny-tiny organisms found inside almost every cell in the human body. They are effectively the power source of a cell and they help to turn the energy from the food we eat into energy that our cells can then use.

The mitochondria in our bodies have their own set of DNA. During conception we get half of our DNA from our father, and the other half from our mother. Interestingly, all of the mitochondrial DNA (mtDNA) we receive at birth – whether we're male or female – can only be passed onwards through the female line, meaning we all inherit this from our mother.

❝ BEFORE WE CAN LOOK AT HOW OUR BODY CHANGES DURING PREGNANCY, AND WHAT WE CAN DO TO HELP IT HEAL, WE NEED TO LOOK AT HOW IT ALL BEGAN. ❞

This makes mtDNA especially useful in tracing back genetic lines. Scientists have found that if we look backwards from mother, back to mother, back to mother, we'd all arrive at one woman, known as Mitochondrial Eve, who roamed the Earth about two hundred thousand years ago.[1]

Let me clarify quickly: Mitochondrial Eve hasn't been discovered as a specific fossil or person. It's the theory itself that was the incredible revelation. This discovery showed that everyone alive on Earth today is a descendant of one homo sapiens woman. This isn't the oldest evidence of all human life on Earth, but where other lines died out, like homo erectus or Neanderthals, the DNA from Mitochondrial Eve still resides in all of us today.

Mitochondrial Eve wouldn't even have been exceptional in her time. There would have been many other women living alongside her. It's possible that other females with this formation of genes even pre-dated or inhabited the Earth alongside her, but something would have caused these lines to be lost.

Modern mothers, bodies and births

So why did I drag you back through this history lesson and what can we, as modern-day mothers, learn from Mitochondrial Eve about how our bodies and minds work today?

The long answer could fill an entire book. The short answer is that we can probably find the roots of everything we do today originating millions of years ago. However, in this chapter I'll keep to the facts relating to pregnancy and motherhood.

Even before Mitochondrial Eve, the female body went through a huge shift in the way it was formed. Humans had gone from walking on four feet (quadrupeds) to standing up on just two (bipeds), and as the years went on, we evolved further apart from our tree-swinging siblings, with the new ability to walk and run on two legs giving us a leg up – excuse the pun – on other mammals at the time.

Learning to walk, and eventually to run, meant that humans were able to travel further afield than other animals. The evidence of certain bones and the development of an arch in our foot shows that we no longer prioritised grasping branches and began to abandon life in the trees, instead travelling across plains by foot to other areas, previously undiscovered by our species.

Eventually homo sapiens, like Mitochondrial Eve, moved their communities to new locations, and the human race spread out in vast populations all over the world.

The act of standing upright also meant that there were huge changes in how women gave birth and it was at this moment that the modern-day pelvic floor began to form.

In the days of walking on all fours, the front of the human abdomen would have been the base of our core and our abdominal muscles would have carried the weight of our growing baby and organs, but once we stood up we needed another support network that could stop things just plopping out at the bottom! So, our tail bone pulled in and – *ta-dah!* – the pelvic floor was created, although probably not with so much pizzazz.

Our pelvis shape and hip width needed to change as well. The female body now had to be able to manage the new skill of walking upright whilst also being able to carry and birth our babies. 'Wide hips' can sometimes be viewed as a complaint for modern-day postnatal women, but we should actually be in awe of this fact. It's Mother Nature doing its incredible work again.

Women had to evolve with a pelvis wide enough to allow babies to grow and be birthed via the birth canal, but narrow enough that it was stable when we stood or needed to move. This is why our pelvis widens during puberty, as our bodies mature enough to be able to withstand pregnancy. This is then enhanced by hormonal changes through the trimesters, which allow our pelvic joints to soften and loosen, creating the space our babies need to be born through the birth canal. Then, during menopause, our pelvis moves back into a narrower form.

All these physical adaptations evolved because of the increased demands that were placed on the female body when humans stood up. Physically, mentally and socially, we operate under very different pressures now. Take the creation of the internet and social media, for example. Although it opened up a new world of communication, it has also meant that many people feel pressured to work longer hours, with more social judgements, often leading to higher levels of stress and expectations to 'do more'.

There seems to be very little time for physical activity, even for something as important as postnatal recovery. Exercise is no longer ingrained in modern humans as a daily necessity. In fact, for many it's seen as an extra-curricular activity, where it was once a part of our everyday life. But as women we shouldn't need to choose between our health and motherhood. We can fit in exercise alongside our other commitments and it's important that we do.

One thing that hasn't changed, though, is that motherhood can be a powerful experience.

When I think back to Mitochondrial Eve birthing the future all those years ago, I feel inspired. She is us! If these original homo sapiens women could create, carry and birth life, with very little support in comparison to the birthing options we have today, then so can we!

Don't misunderstand me: as a mother myself I am well aware of the challenges we can face during pregnancy and postpartum. But the fact remains, we do all still have what it takes to thrive during this period. It's literally in our DNA.

However we dress, whatever we look like, we are all linked to the Eves that came before us. We have the foundations. Now it's up to us to build on them and truly become **StrongLikeMum**.

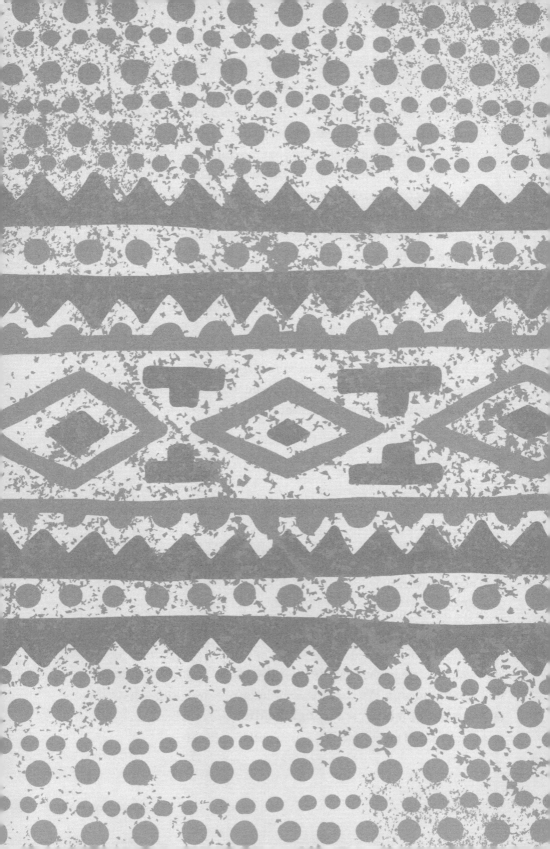

Mind over muscle

We've all been there, those long nights when your baby decides sleep is for suckers or when you encounter a poop so colossal it somehow makes its way into sleeves and down trouser legs. Motherhood doesn't come with a manual and largely we rely on our instinct to teach us how to raise a baby. Indeed, when a poo-nami hits, it's down to us to find a way of successfully tidying it up with minimal damage to baby, clothes, carpet and ourselves.

But pre- and postnatal fitness doesn't need to be such a solo venture. Sometimes a little support can be the difference between simply surviving and thriving.

For a long time, finding advice on pre- and postnatal fitness was like searching for a needle in a haystack, but now it seems as though the scale is tipping in the opposite direction towards information overload. The internet is littered with an abundance of contradictory information, and old-school myths are sprawled across the web. This barrage of misinformation has led to mass confusion about how to safely and successfully rehabilitate our bodies.

Perhaps it's because we've moved away from natural remedies and live in a society where 'quick fixes' are desirable. At a time when coffee is instant, TV is on demand and wifi is super-fast, we seem to have lost sight of how and why we should create slower yet more sustainable processes. Knowing how to safely rehabilitate our bodies postnatally isn't a quick fix. It takes some groundwork in order to lay strong foundations and help our bodies cope with future loads.

This is why, before we focus on building our biceps, we need to build self-belief, so that we can create a deep-rooted connection to our body that no bad mood can break.

This begins with words: the words we use, those we surround ourselves with and, most importantly, those we allow to settle in!

The word cycle

There is a problem in the fitness industry and it needs fixing, quickly. It's the way new mothers are bombarded with unrealistic phrases and negative language. ALL. THE. TIME.

I first noticed this at a gym I worked in, back in 2013. A poster on the wall claimed women could 'bounce back' from pregnancy to achieve their summer body goals. After all these years, working in pre- and postnatal health and after becoming a mother myself four times over, I can officially confirm that 'bounce back' is an illusion.

It does not exist. Nor should it!

Pregnancy is a 10-month journey full of physical and hormonal changes. The entire process culminates in an intense effort during labour, which brings to the world a brand new life. The idea of 'bouncing back' after that does not sound safe to me. I can't stress enough the importance of laying stable foundations in the postnatal period. By creating stability in the deep core of our body, we can ensure that we're able to support more strenuous movements later on.

Unfortunately, it seems as though we haven't progressed much in the last few years with the kind of language we use. I still hear trainers claiming women can get their 'pre-baby body back' or 'drop a dress size' quickly after pregnancy. Not only are these terms unrealistic, they are unachievable and, to be frank, ridiculous!

We shouldn't be 'snapping back' at all. By using these phrases, we are paving the way for a dangerous mindset, allowing stereotypes to determine how all mothers should be feeling after birth.

I read a paper published in *Psychological Science,* which suggests that the language we use can directly impact our ability to perform a task or achieve a goal.[2] This is why The **StrongLikeMum** Method begins not with sit-ups or circuits, but by looking at the impact affirmations can have on our pre- and postnatal fitness journey. These then become part of our daily routine, and they are just as important as the right exercise and diet choices.

We are constantly surrounded by words, from the TV we watch to the music we listen to and even the people we hang out with or the way we speak about ourselves. Historically, women were discouraged from supporting one another to be heard, but the tide is changing now. From Emmeline Pankhurst to the Beyoncés and Sheryl Sandbergs of the world, in many places the female empowerment movement is well on its way.

How can we join the movement? I believe it stems from the word cycle:

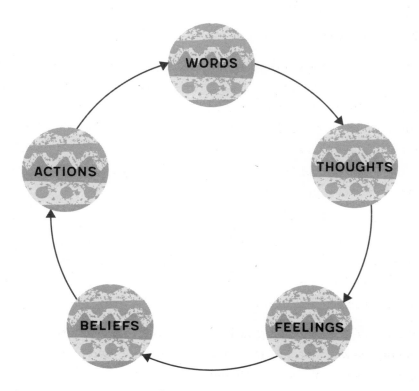

This word cycle demonstrates how our words can affect our beliefs and thereby our actions. The words we use on a regular basis begin to influence our thoughts. Repetitive thoughts begin to inspire feelings and it's our feelings that form the basis of our beliefs. Finally, our beliefs begin to determine how we act on a regular basis. If the words we use encourage insecurity on a base level, it's no surprise they can develop into self-doubt and uncertainty.

If we've been absorbing the damaging rhetoric of bounce-back over many, many years, we need to counteract this by focusing on creating a positive word cycle for ourselves.

It's time to rebel against negative habits. Just as we can edit our Instagram feed and 'unfollow' a Facebook page, we can also curate our life feed. We can use words to inspire us and boost our confidence and self-belief, much like prenatal women do when using hypnobirthing mantras.

From there we will be able to build our physical goals, with a firmer base to help us maintain any changes.

Don't worry if this thought is daunting; this is what this chapter is going to help with and using positive words is the crucial first step.

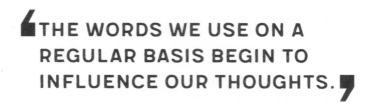

THE WORDS WE USE ON A REGULAR BASIS BEGIN TO INFLUENCE OUR THOUGHTS.

Affirmations, mantras and visualisation

Let me start with a note for any cynics. If you're feeling like you might just skip the rest of this chapter, thinking 'mantras are for hippies', I ask that you hold off from making any snap judgements for a moment and give it a chance. I'm convinced that by the end you'll soon see that we can't achieve whole-body health without tapping into the power of our mind.

When it comes to birth, our mindset is crucial. And for recently postnatal women, how we feel directly impacts our recovery. For example, if you have given birth via a caesarean section, research shows that emotional stress can trigger scar tissue regrowth, which can bind itself around other organs or internal body tissue.[3] So we really should prioritise ways to stay positive and relieve stress.

And it's not only relevant for the immediate postnatal period. Our state of mind can impact all of our parenting, from simple, everyday tasks to staying calm in moments of chaos. In my opinion, mental health is as important as physical fitness.

When it comes to mantras more specifically, there are many times we use them daily, even without realising it. I'm sure most parents can relate to repeating 'stay awake' or 'stay calm' during a night feed after what feels like the hundredth wake-up!

But what of the cynics who are still eye-rolling this entire page, sceptical about whether the use of mantras actually has any effect?

I had this debate recently with my husband, who, while not necessarily a cynic, is certainly a realist who prefers to deal in facts.

It was a rainy Saturday afternoon, and his attention was torn between building Lego with our children and a football match on TV between Portsmouth and Hull.

'Come on Pompey,' he shouted. 'We can do this!'

'Ha!' I said, with perhaps a teensy bit of smugness. 'That's a mantra right there.'

Because mantras, I was happy to point out to my husband, aren't just for those who consider themselves deeply spiritual; a mantra is a statement, repeated out loud, with the intention of inspiring a result. Chants and verses, whether said internally or shouted at a sports team, are all a form of mantra.

If it helps, we can remove the word 'mantra' and instead refer to it as self-talk.

No such thing as negative?

I had an insightful chat with a friend about this recently – psychologist, author and mother Anna Mathur (@annamathur). 'Mantras are a form of self-talk,' she told me. 'The key is in changing your internal dialogue to create a positive narrative.'

Anna made it clear, though, that we can't ignore our negative emotions when we have them.

'Feeling upset or irritated is a natural part of human nature,' Anna explained. 'And ignoring this can actually make more stress and negative emotions build up. If they're left unaddressed, they will grow, not dwindle. No one can be expected to feel great all of the time. And it's important that we don't invalidate some of our feelings.'

Anna pointed out that coping and moving on from negative emotions helps our brain to realise that we have what it takes to adjust and recover. It's in the act of processing what we feel that we can learn to accept and then move on, knowing next time we will be wiser and more prepared.

'We do want to make sure that we're not wallowing in negative thoughts though,' Anna cautioned. 'Whilst it's one thing to blow off steam, cry, shout or rant in frustration, we should then prioritise finding a way back into a positive mindset.'

I thought about this a lot on the way home. If Anna was right, and we need to be able to recognise our challenges without becoming over-whelmed by them, then what a successful mantra should do is not cover up our insecurities, but change how we perceive them and remind us that we *can* cope.

When it comes to fitness, especially as it relates to pregnancy health and postnatal recovery, our mantras should remind us of our inherent female power.

Maybe we could learn a thing or two from the self-talk we encourage our children to have. We teach them to believe that anything is possible if they work hard enough. Should they fail, we teach them that it's okay to slip up and they must try again. We speak to them with patience and kindness and positive language. Maybe we'd benefit from nurturing ourselves a little like this too.

❛BECAUSE MANTRAS AREN'T JUST FOR THOSE WHO CONSIDER THEMSELVES DEEPLY SPIRITUAL; A MANTRA IS A STATEMENT, REPEATED OUT LOUD, WITH THE INTENTION OF INSPIRING A RESULT.❜

Making a mantra

There is no one way to create a mantra. However, the phrase must resonate with a positive feeling, and we should try to keep mantras in the present tense too, as we are dealing in the now. The aim is for your brain to link your future goals with your current state of being.

This is how I create them for myself:

Acknowledge
Realise
Imagine
Sync
Exhale

Step 1: Acknowledge

We always need to acknowledge our starting point, which will be different for us all. We cannot compare ourselves to others.

To create a mantra, start by identifying an area where you feel challenged and want to improve. This may make you feel vulnerable, but acknowledging and accepting our struggles is key. As we overcome them, we will build strength.

Try to be specific and avoid using words that bring you down, even if they are the first ones that come to mind. If you feel 'my stomach's bloated', try to go a level deeper than the immediate emotion. You might want to journal a short paragraph about how you're feeling or, if you're pressed for time, try to find three substitute words or phrases that convey the same message. Maybe something like: 'I want to tone and strengthen my core.'

Step 2: Realise

Now that we've acknowledged an area we'd like to improve, let's briefly think about the tools we already have to get our goal.

For example, 'I am learning what I need to progress' or 'I have the determination to persevere'.

Step 3: Imagine

Put yourself in the mindset of having achieved your goal. Visualisation is the key to making mantras work. Allow yourself to feel the emotions and pride at completing your goal. Drink in the sensation. What does it feel like? 'I am proud of my achievement.'

Step 4: Sync

Now link the three elements together into one long sentence.

For example, 'I want to strengthen my core, I have what it takes to persevere and I am proud of my achievement.'

Step 5: Exhale

Take a deep inhale and, on the exhale, release any negative feelings around the first part of the sentence. We're going to delete it!

Once we release the first part of the sentence, we have our mantra!

'I have what it takes to persevere and I am proud of myself.'

Now we put it into practice. Every day! Start the day with some positive self-talk. Fuel your body with a positive mindset and see how your actions are changed as a result.

As we move through the rest of this book and rehabilitate our bodies, keep this in the forefront of your mind. If we approach our pregnancy fitness and postnatal recovery with this mindset, we can maintain any positive changes with truly strong, powerful and unbreakable foundations.

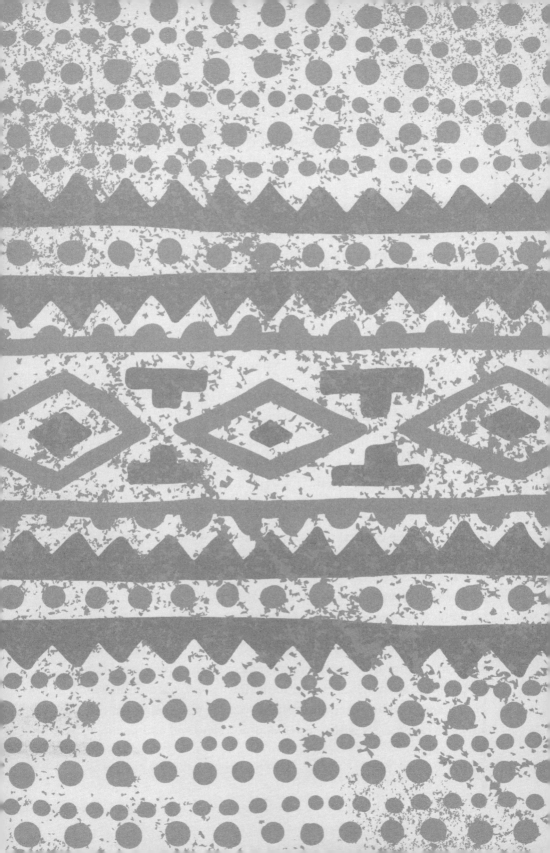

Basics of the female core

Before starting on which exercises are best and how to do them, I wanted to share a few insights into the basis of the female core. Having clarity around how things change in our body during pregnancy gives us an understanding of why our body needs foundation movements before progressing to faster, more intense exercises.

Without wanting to state the glaringly obvious, pregnancy, labour and birth are no walk in the park. In fact, it's said that pregnancy demands the same energy expenditure as running a 40-day marathon[4] and the process of labour can be as taxing on the body as extreme endurance exercise, like running 26 miles![5]

The idea of completing either of these feats without training isn't feasible. So never again should we question whether exercise in pregnancy is safe, because not only is it safe, it's needed!

The difference between running a marathon and giving birth, aside from the human 'popping' out of you, is that post-marathon runners can usually drop to the floor in exhaustion, soak in a bath for a few hours and have a good uninterrupted rest. I'm not sure about others, but the arrival of my children certainly wasn't met with the same tranquillity.

Pregnancy, labour and birth are hugely demanding for our entire body. But arguably the biggest impact is to our core. That's not to say that other areas of the body aren't affected; in fact it's the opposite, because when our core is affected, everything else is too!

bigger than you might think. It's not simply made up
...ominal (stomach) muscles. There's also the pelvic floor, glutes,
abductor, adductor (thigh) and lower back muscles working too.
Together this entire network of muscles makes up our complete core,
and they are the starting block for *all* our bodily movements.

Let's take a quick dive into our core so we can understand how it's
connected to the rest of our body and mind. Then, when we come to
exercise, we'll know why each movement is important and how it
supports a healthy pregnancy and post-birth recovery.

I promise to keep this interesting and not to turn it into a GCSE anatomy
textbook!

Pelvic power

At the very base of our core is our pelvic floor which, as we know, evolved
over a very long period of time.

In the current set-up, our pelvic floor muscles are positioned almost like
a hammock at the base of our torso. This relatively small muscle group
carries a huge amount of pressure even before pregnancy: supporting all
our internal organs, helping with functions like bladder and bowel
control, and providing passage for our urethra, vagina and rectum.
When the extra weight of baby, placenta and amniotic fluid is added
on top during pregnancy, it's no wonder these muscles get tired, or
unbalanced.

The thought that pelvic floor health was left largely neglected by the
fitness industry until recent years is tragic. Kegel exercises were
probably the only exercise spoken about, but this only scratches the
surface of what's really needed for an efficient recovery and doesn't at all
share with women the details of what happens to their body during and
after pregnancy! In the twenty-first century the discussion around
pelvic floor health has thankfully opened up, but there's still a long way
to go in making this information accessible to everyone. Hopefully this
is the start.

Evolutionarily speaking, the female body had to make a compromise in terms of our pelvic region. We needed a narrow enough pelvis for stable movement but a wide enough space for pregnancy and birth. And the ingenuity of Mother Nature didn't stop there.

The design of the female body works perfectly alongside the development of our babies in utero. For example, at the time of birth a fully developed human brain would need a much bigger head circumference than our narrow pelvis could handle.

This is why a newborn baby's skull is soft and flexible, designed with gaps between the plates of bone. These plates can shift across one another, allowing the circumference of our baby's head to decrease during delivery. If the brain was to grow much more in utero, it could make vaginal delivery dangerous even with the shifting plates at work.

For humans, the development to an adult-sized brain happens mostly outside of the womb. The process to maturity takes longer than many other animals, but it's also a more advanced process. Take a foal, for example, that can stand up within just a few hours of birth. Humans often take a year or more to master this skill.

> **EVOLUTIONARILY SPEAKING, THE FEMALE BODY HAD TO MAKE A COMPROMISE IN TERMS OF OUR PELVIC REGION. WE NEEDED A NARROW ENOUGH PELVIS FOR STABLE MOVEMENT BUT A WIDE ENOUGH SPACE FOR PREGNANCY AND BIRTH.**

If humans were born at an equal maturity to horses or even baby monkeys – who can cling to their mother from birth and are fully independent between two and four years old – we would need to remain in utero for up to 21 months. That's an entire year longer than the average human gestation period.

It's clear to see that nature and evolution created amazing coping strategies to preserve the birthing process for us humans, while still keeping the female body mobile and strong. Nonetheless our pelvic floor and the wider structure of the female body have to work harder to support our core as we move through pregnancy and onwards into a mobile motherhood.

Fortunately, our pelvic floor isn't working alone. It has the support of our entire core to keep us active and strong. Our glutes, lower back, upper legs, abdominals and respiratory system all team together.

How is your pelvic floor linked to the rest of your body?

Your core is connected to the rest of your body by a thin layer of body tissue known as myofascia.

In a nutshell, there are two types of fascia: superficial and deep. Superficial fascia is found just under our skin and acts as a storage system for fat and water. Deep myofascia, on the other hand, is a strong web of body tissue that connects all our muscles, tendons, ligaments, nerves and bones, like a whole body suit that runs from the top of our head to the tips of our toes. Fascia is designed to be strong but stretch when we move.

Myofascia is one of those technical terms that is rarely spoken about outside of the fitness industry, but everyone should be aware of it as it surrounds all of our muscles and plays a key role in holding our entire frame together.

Okay, I'm starting to sound like that GCSE textbook I was trying to avoid. Basically, every time our body completes a task like reaching, bending, walking or balancing, our myofascia is helping the process by keeping everything connected and working together.

Thomas Myers, a leading integrative manual therapist, talks about multiple 'lines' of myofascia that run through the body. Picture a map of the London Underground, with each line running in a different direction to a different area of the body. Arms, legs, neck and so on.

Try tracing the deep front line with your finger as you read, for an insight into the connection between the pelvic floor and the rest of your body.

The line most relevant to pre- and postnatal health is called the myofascial deep front line (DFL) which runs from the bottom of our foot, behind our knee, via the pelvis, pelvic floor and core, through the ribcage, rising up our neck and passing through our jaw, ending either side of our skull.

The DFL is shifted out of optimal alignment as pregnancy progresses and our posture changes. For example, as our pregnancy bump grows, the position of our pelvis is tilted forwards and, as a result, the DFL is pulled out of alignment.

After pregnancy our aim with exercise should be to realign this network, with exercise and posture. If any changes are left unresolved, it means we could begin to form damaging habits with our movements that can lead to pain or injury later on in life.

So often I've had women come to me years after pregnancy complaining of knee pain or lower back ache and, after investigating, more often than not, the trigger can be found somewhere along the deep front line.

As this line is quite long, pinpointing something along the way that needs our attention takes time, but at least we have a guide on where to start looking.

Just becoming aware of how much tension we're holding in this area is a good place to start.

Have you ever noticed that you are clenching your jaw, curling your toes or rolling to the outsides of your feet? All of these areas are connected to our pelvic floor, meaning that they can be symptoms of dysfunction along the DFL, and this can have an effect on your pelvic floor.

After having my twins, I noticed pretty quickly that I was clenching my jaw a lot. I had birthed via a caesarean section this time, so wasn't anticipating tension in the pelvic floor area, but I soon realised that this 'gripping' I was doing was due to the caesarean incision. My body was trying to re-establish balance when the wound was still healing, and I was feeling the repercussions far from the trigger point. It works in reverse too. We might clench our jaw, in frustration or concentration and, as a result, our pelvic floor can become tense too.

Being aware of the connection from our pelvic floor to the rest of the body should encourage us to work on whole body health, rather than just isolated recovery. The pelvic floor is literally the centre of all our body movements.

❝SO OFTEN I'VE HAD WOMEN COME TO ME WELL AFTER PREGNANCY COMPLAINING OF KNEE PAIN OR BACK ACHE AND, AFTER INVESTIGATING, MORE OFTEN THAN NOT, THE TRIGGER IS FROM SOMEWHERE ALONG THE DEEP FRONT LINE.❞

DFL body scan exercise

- Lie on your back on a flat surface. If you're prenatal you may wish to do this seated or even standing against a wall.

- Take a few deep breaths, keeping your shoulders relaxed and arms relaxed by your sides.

- If you're lying down, your legs should be extended along the floor.

- Keep your breathing steady and slow.

- With each inhale focus on a specific body part, starting with your toes. Inhale and on the exhale release any tension.

- Focus first on the toes, then your ankles, calves, knees, thighs, pelvic floor, glutes, hips, spine, chest, shoulders, neck, tongue, cheeks.

- Once the scan is complete relax for a few minutes and turn your attention to the path of the DFL. Do you notice any differences? Were you holding any excess tension along this line?

- You may wish to repeat the scan a second time and notice if any tension has built up again without you realising.

Pelvic energy in pregnancy and postpartum

We can't talk about the pelvic floor without going a little deeper into how it functions. Because the role of the pelvic floor doesn't stop with movements. Many believe its true power runs even deeper, because our pelvic floor is also home to our energy system.

Energy fluctuation seems to be a theme throughout pregnancy and parenthood. We can be supercharged one day and feel as though we're snail-pacing the next.

With our hormone levels continually changing, it makes sense that our emotions and energy levels will fluctuate too.

Interestingly some women notice a big energy boost at the start of pregnancy. It's not yet confirmed why, but evidence suggests it's due to the increase in the amount of blood in our system, as our body prepares to support the growth of our embryo in utero.

Ever noticed that you're much thirstier when you become pregnant? Well, that is also thought to be due to the increase in the amount of blood in our body after conception. We need the water to help support the increasing levels of blood supply.

This rise in blood volume also means more blood flows through our blood vessels at any given time, leaving our skin looking flushed and glowing, which is where the term 'pregnancy glow' comes from. Alongside all of this, the size of our heart is also thought to increase in early pregnancy, to help with the extra demand from the increased levels of blood. Combined, all of these factors are thought to give a significant boost to our cardiovascular fitness, therefore boosting energy!

Unfortunately, not everyone experiences raging energy surges at this time. For some, this potential energy spike is masked by the arrival of morning sickness, which can drain our energy as fast as we acquire it. This up-and-down energy dance continues throughout the entire prenatal period, and from then on, it seems, motherhood can be a non-stop energy rollercoaster. But it turns out that our pelvic floor health might just be the key to unlocking stores of untapped energy.

Both modern science and ancient spirituality agree that maintaining good energy levels improves our overall health and speeds up the rate of recovery. Whether you buy into spiritual metaphors or not, the theory is simple: by letting go of physical tensions and releasing emotional stress, we can allow more energy to flow, assisting recovery.

How is any of this relevant to pelvic floor health? Well, energy balance takes place via our chakra line which is intrinsically connected to our pelvic health.

What have chakras got to do with your core?

Although I'm no expert on chakras, I want to share a snippet of what I do know.

There are seven 'main' chakras located along our spine, and they are believed to be among hundreds of others located throughout the body. Many believe that when the energy flowing along this line is balanced, our body can move freely, without tension.

Two of the main chakras are located close to the pelvic floor. The first of seven in the tantric energy system is the root chakra. (And for any filth-pots reading, tantra is not just about sex!) The word *tantra* comes from Sanskrit and refers to the idea that everyone and everything is interconnected, the human body being the perfect example.

According to ancient Eastern traditions, the root chakra – also known as 'The Muladhara' – is situated at our coccyx. As the name suggests, the root chakra is the base of all our energy. Like the roots of a tree it works almost like a portal, helping to keep us grounded, drawing up energy like water to keep us nourished and strong.

This is followed slightly further up the spine by the sacral chakra – also known as 'Svadhishthana' – which is found about four to five fingers' width above the first, just below the line of your belly button. Remember, the chakra line moves along the spine and not up the front of the body.

Spine mobility is a hugely underrated element of exercise. Moving our spine and, by extension, our body allows us to keep these chakras open. If you're pregnant, the mobility of your spine will affect how you feel as pregnancy progresses and your bump begins to grow. Your entire centre of gravity changes, and your spine and core need to adapt to manage the new load.

For some reason, many people only pay attention to their spine health in retrospect; not until they feel a stiff neck or suffer with back pain does the mobility of their spine become a priority. But particularly for pre- and postnatal women, we should remember to mobilise our spine.

I should say here that back bends are a controversial movement in pregnancy, because of the pressure they may create on the front of our abdominal wall, especially in the second and third trimesters as well as immediately postpartum. At these times we're better served focusing on a neutral spine or bending forwards (spinal flexion). Small extensions can be okay in exercises like the cat-cow position but this should be more a subtle tilt of the pelvis, rather than a deliberate arching of the back.

Both Mudlahara and Svadhishthana are associated with physical touchpoints on the body. Places we can feel that are strongly linked to pelvic health.

Spiritually, a balanced root chakra is thought to encourage feelings of security, calm and being grounded. The second chakra, Svadhishthana, is often associated with the ovaries in women, or testes in men, and is said to influence relationships, sexual behaviours and reproduction.

To unblock these chakras, ancient traditions call for what we in the present day call pelvic health exercises.

The premise is simple: we need good alignment, physically and emotionally, to establish harmony in our deep core, and by using a combination of pelvic floor exercises, breath work, meditation and mindfulness, we can establish balance.

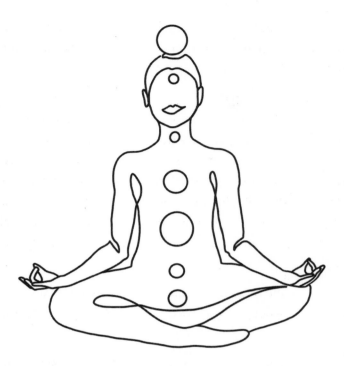

From spirituality to *Friends*

Pelvic floor exercises are actually simple movements, but it's so important that we do them correctly and activate our whole pelvic floor as opposed to only a few muscles.

The best example I can give as to why is through an old TV series that was popular in my teens called *Friends*. One famous scene sees the characters trying to lift a couch up a flight of steps, attempting multiple techniques to pivot the sofa into place. But with a mismatch of strengths between the characters, the sofa falls over the banister.

Let's imagine that this sofa is our pelvic floor and the friends supporting it are the surrounding muscles and ligaments, like our glutes and lower back.

If everyone lifts together, with equal strength, the sofa can be lifted off the floor. But if one friend is weaker than the others, they will all struggle equally to support the couch, and the weaker member will bear the brunt even more.

Similarly, if one of the friends is working too hard (is overactive) and puts too much force behind the lift, the weight of the sofa will again be shifted onto the other supporters, who could falter and break down under the pressure.

Equal balance is needed from all muscles to support the core properly. Exercises can help us to create a balance in our core and this balance begins with our breath.

Belly breathing

By using our breath well, we can enhance the ability of our core to work properly. Good core control will help us rectify imbalances that might have sprung up along the DFL during pregnancy.

People spend so much time crunching and planking to get good abs, when in actual fact, if we really want a strong core, what we should be doing is slowing down and practising a good breath first.

'Diaphragmatic breathing', or 'belly breathing', have become buzz words over the years, but what exactly do they mean?

Belly breathing is a technique that engages our diaphragm, a muscle that sits underneath our ribs and helps us take a better breath.

This muscle is dome-shaped and moves up and down, a bit like a parachute filling with air. If you imagine attaching a parachute in the middle of a circle of trees, then stretching it out, that's similar to how our diaphragm is positioned.

As we inhale and draw air in on top of the diaphragm the parachute fills with air, the middle dropping downwards. As we exhale, the air is pushed up and out and the parachute lifts up again.

The act of breathing is so natural that many of us take it for granted, never considering it as anything other than a regular – although very necessary – daily function. But, as natural as breathing may be, doing it properly is an art many adults seem to have lost.

When we breathe in, and our diaphragm – the parachute – fills and moves downwards, all our organs underneath need to move down a bit as well. If our pelvic floor is relaxed, we have more space for this to happen. Then, when we exhale, we will have more power in our core to work with.

Our diaphragm is essential for optimal breath work, and plays a key role in synchronising the core muscles to work alongside each other, allowing us to reset our pelvic alignment.

Breathing well takes focus and control and is so powerful when done correctly. Here's how …

Meet your TPC

Here's the last piece of the puzzle when learning how to breathe correctly. Let me introduce you to your thoracic pelvic cylinder. Sounds sexy, right?

Like your deep core, your thoracic pelvic cylinder (TPC) is composed of many muscle groups, although this time it's not just the lower region that's involved. Your TPC is the area of your body that runs from your first rib all the way down to your pelvic floor. It's essentially the mid-section of the DFL.

THE THORACIC PELVIC CYLINDER

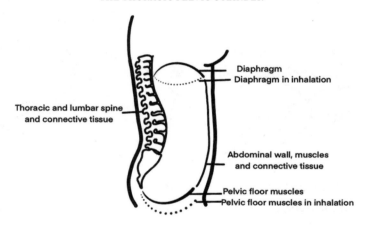

Your TPC includes your pelvic floor, glutes, adductors, abductors, hip flexors, lower back, thorax, inner organs, diaphragm, lungs, rib cage and chest.

To take a 'proper' breath, we must fill this entire region. Our shoulders should remain down and relaxed. Our rib cage expands outwards and the diaphragm descends. Our breath should be felt through 360 degrees, from the top of the TPC (ribcage) and down to the pelvic floor, along the front and rear abdominal walls, as well as sideways, as our rib cage expands.

Simply put, shoulders down, ribs out and pelvic floor relaxed. We can practise this with the exercise below.

Three-dimensional breathing exercise

This exercise can be used by pre- or postnatal women; however, for anyone over 16 weeks gestation, the current NHS guidelines state that pregnant women should avoid lying on their backs for long periods of time. In this case, we can do this exercise siting on a chair, feet flat on the floor, hip-width apart.

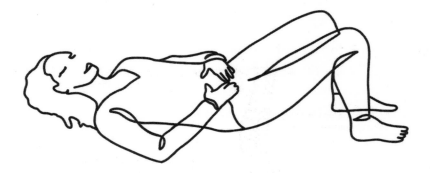

● Lie back on the floor in the semi-supine position, meaning your feet are flat on the floor, knees bent up, keeping your legs hip-width apart. You may also choose to support your head with a soft block or pillow.

● As we breathe in we want to initiate the three dimensions, which are:
    1 Expansion of the rib cage;
    2 Feeling the air fill your torso by the sensation of connecting your back with the floor;
    3 Relaxation of the pelvic floor.

● Close your eyes and as you inhale, imagine the three stages taking place. Imagine the ribcage expanding, back connecting with the floor and pelvic floor muscles relaxing.

● Remember to keep your shoulders relaxed. If you notice them lifting, it's a sign that you're not inhaling fully so relax and start again.

● With each subsequent inhale, visualise relaxing your pelvic floor muscles to create more space for your breath. A relaxed floor gives your organs more space to move downwards as the lungs fill up and the diaphragm descends.

● You may wish to place your hands low down on your belly, just above your pubic bone, to feel your belly filling with each inhale.

● Exhale slowly for a count of eight. As you do so, draw up your pelvic floor by visualising your coccyx bone at the back and pubic bone at the front coming together and lifting up. This will encourage complete activation of our pelvic floor (more details on p.149).

● Inhale and release. Repeat this exercise for a few minutes.

● Stay aware of an increase in movement and mobilisation within your thorax (chest) as you breathe in.

● You should be able to fully relax your pelvic floor on the inhale, but without the sensation of pushing or bearing down. Focus on release and relaxation with each 'in' breath.

The experts

As with most exercise techniques, there are industry leaders paving the way and setting good examples. In the world of breathing there are many such gurus . . . we call them babies!

Have you ever said your baby has a 'Buddha belly'? Well, this endearing term is not without reason; babies are the world's leading experts in diaphragmatic breathing.

It's a bit frustrating to realise that we all had it right to begin with, but we managed to mess things up as we aged. Whether due to emotional stress or muscular tensions, the majority of us adults have moved away from the way we used to breathe as babies.

If you watch your baby breathe, you will see their belly expand, filling like a balloon, with their shoulders relaxed and, although you might not notice it, their diaphragm is also descending.

Babies know how to breathe right, sit with perfect posture and maintain alignment when they come to standing. Granted, their standing efforts are often followed by core imbalance and a fall, but still, they get a ten out of ten for posture!

HAVE YOU EVER SAID YOUR BABY HAS A "BUDDHA BELLY"? WELL, THIS ENDEARING TERM IS NOT WITHOUT REASON; BABIES ARE THE WORLD'S LEADING EXPERTS IN DIAPHRAGMATIC BREATHING.

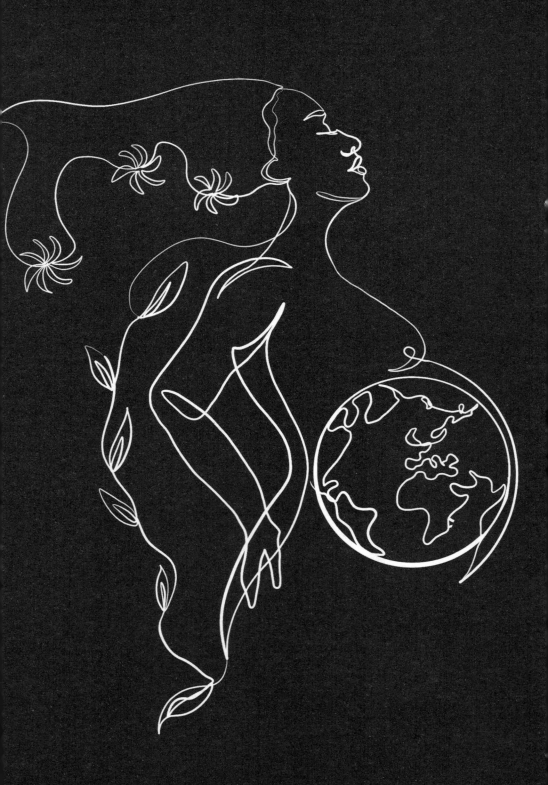

POWER

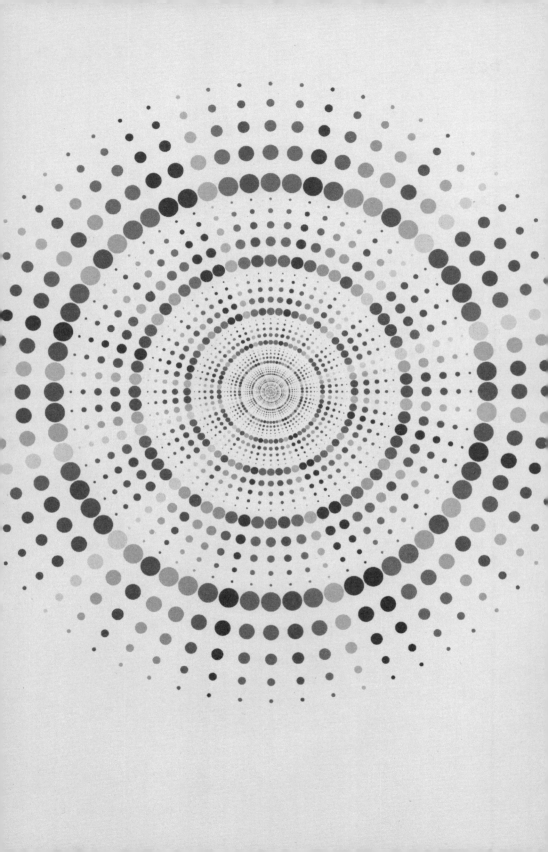

Physicality in pregnancy

I'm aware that each of you reading this book will be coming at it from different perspectives. Some of you might be reading this during your first pregnancy. Or you might have already given birth. Maybe you are an experienced mother who welcomed your baby many moons ago.

Regardless of where you are on the journey, knowing the changes we go through in pregnancy is important, even long after we are considered postnatal, because it can give us an insight into why we're feeling certain things now.

I'd also recommend ear-marking this chapter. You might just find that you come back to it in a subsequent pregnancy and absorb completely different points to those you take away today.

The core shift

Our body goes through so many changes in pregnancy but let's start with the shift in our core. Prior to pregnancy, a healthy functioning core means that all our deep core muscles, like our pelvic floor and transverse abdominis, work together with the other surrounding core muscles, like our glutes and lower back, to help us lift, carry, rotate, jump and run. They all work in synergy.

In pregnancy, however, the alignment of our core is altered. For example, as the trimesters progress our pelvis is tilted forwards, in order to allow our uterus to expand, making space for our baby (or babies) to grow and our bump to get bigger. This pelvic tilt happens in all pregnancies and is a natural part of the process.

If you stand in front of a mirror you can test this out and see the ripple effect for yourself.

PRIOR TO PREGNANCY, A HEALTHY FUNCTIONING CORE MEANS THAT ALL OUR DEEP CORE MUSCLES, LIKE OUR PELVIC FLOOR AND TRANSVERSE ABDOMINIS, WORK TOGETHER WITH THE OTHER SURROUNDING CORE MUSCLES...

Pelvic tilt during pregnancy

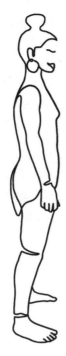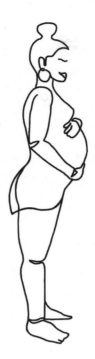

Stand side-on to a mirror, place your hands on your hips and imagine a pregnancy bump – or maybe you don't need to imagine. As the weight of the baby and uterus increases and your bump grows outwards, your pelvis is tilted forwards and an arch is expressed in your lower back. You might begin to notice that your bottom starts to stick out behind you more. This posture is referred to as lordosis. This can lead to a tightness and crunching sensation in your lower back as well as placing increased pressure on the front of your abdominal wall.

It might seem like a tiny shift, but over time this tilt of your pelvis and arch of your lower back could mean that your internal organs are forced to rest slightly off the bony structures of your pelvis, placing increased pressure on your pelvic floor.

Don't worry! Our body is designed to manage these changes in pregnancy, and although we can't stop this tilt from happening, we can work on supporting the surrounding core muscles to create stability.

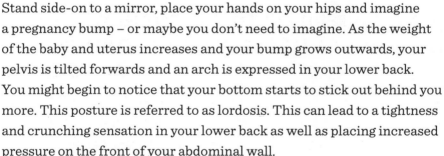

When it comes to the pelvic tilt, our pelvis will usually settle back into its original position by 6 months postpartum, all on its own. However, we want to make sure that we continue to keep any eye on our posture even after this time. We might find we've adopted some bad habits that could have a detrimental effect if left over time and might seem tricky to change even long after we've given birth.

Honestly, it never fails to amaze me how such a simple shift during pregnancy can be the cause of so many physical complaints, even years later. I've worked with countless women who have been suffering with knee pain, or have tight calves, or pronate when they walk (landing on the outer edges of their feet), and are unsure why. After some work together we've come to realise that it's all been down to not addressing pelvic realignment after pregnancy.

But as I said, don't panic, it's not all doom and gloom; the good news is that it's never too late to begin working on posture and core stability. If we address the root cause, we can stop this cycle. By correcting our foundations we can reverse damaging habits and alleviate many related symptoms and pain.

I'll be sharing lots of exercises to help manage this shift in this chapter. However, there are, of course, many other changes happening in our body during pregnancy too. So let's look at some other ripple effects and the impact they can have on us physically.

Baby bump

I was so excited when I saw the beginnings of my first baby bump.
I remember feeling as though I had to wait ages for it to show up, pushing
out my tummy at parties hoping someone might ask whether I was
carrying and join in my excitement in the run-up to the birth. At twenty-
three years old, I had only been training women for a few years and it
hadn't yet occurred to me just how much my growing bump could
impact the rest of my body.

Alongside initiating a tilt of our pelvis, the increasing size of our uterus
places pressure on the front of our abdominal wall.

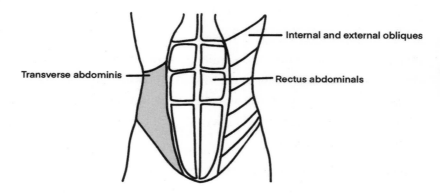

Did you know that your abs are split into four layers? The deepest of
these is called the transverse abdominis (TVA), which lies underneath
all our other abdominal muscles. Together with our back muscles, the
TVA works like a wrap-around, 'hugging' our spinal column and torso
to keep us supported.

When we hold any static contraction, like a plank, the TVA engages to
keep our torso stable. Imagine an olden-day Elizabethan corset being
pulled tight. When our TVA contracts, it acts in a similar way to this.
To activate it, inhale and then blow out air as if you're blowing out a
candle – that sharp pull in is your TVA at work.

When we're pregnant, it's mostly exercises that gently target the TVA
that are recommended for core training.

On top of this are the internal and external obliques. Both of these muscle groups lie diagonally across our torso, over the TVA. Their primary role is to assist with movements where we need to rotate.

Finally, we have the rectus abdominis muscle, which, in my opinion, has been hogging centre stage for years. It's the 'six pack' muscle and is the outermost layer of our abdominal four. The rectus abdominis muscle has commanded the spotlight for a long time, but just as a top goal scorer needs their team in order to achieve success, so does the rectus abdominis need the rest of our core to function properly.

As our bump grows, the two halves of our rectus abdominis muscle move out to the side. Although the muscles separate, contrary to popular belief, there is no tearing or splitting of the muscle itself. This separation actually happens via a length of fascia called the linea alba, which runs vertically along the mid-line, between the two halves of the rectus abdominis muscle. It's the linea alba that stretches as our bump grows, moving our rectus abdominis muscles out to the sides.

If you consider how pregnancy progresses, it's no surprise that there is a weakening of the front of our abdomen. Our once tough muscular abdominal wall has been compromised by the widened linea alba, which although strong itself, needs careful management when we're exercising.

Diastasis recti

Diastasis recti is the official name given to this separation of the rectus abdominis muscle. One hundred per cent of women who reach full term will experience diastasis recti during pregnancy. It's a natural process and, just like the pelvic shift, it's necessary to make space for our baby and bump to grow.

After birth, the gap between the two halves of the rectus abdominis muscle will largely come back together on its own, without needing any assistance. However, for 60 per cent of new mums a small gap may persist after the 8–12-week check, and for some women, the gap never completely closes.

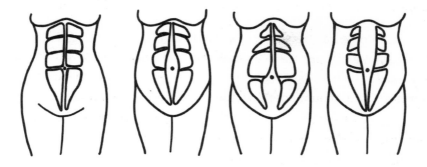

No diastasis   Open Diastasis   Open below the navel   Open above the navel

If you're diagnosed with diastasis recti after 8 weeks postpartum, there's no need to immediately worry. There are lots of exercises we can use to heal this separation, or if like me, you have a small gap that never completely closes, there are exercises to help create a strong core, even without complete closure.

We'll look at postnatal recovery exercises in chapters 9, 10 and 15, but to make sure we still have an efficient core during and after pregnancy we want to prioritise movements that primarily target our TVA, like the exercises coming up, and those recommended in the chapters on exercise throughout the trimesters. It's important that we avoid over-stressing our rectus abdominis muscle with traditional ab exercises like crunches or sit-ups, instead using the TVA and core support muscles as our body adapts in pregnancy.

Interestingly, for women with diastasis recti, the way our obliques are performing is also important. It's not often spoken about, but in the picture of our abdominal layers on page 49 we can see that our obliques have an attachment point leading to the linea alba. If our obliques are too tight, they can pull on these attachment points at either side and actually restrict the gap from coming together.

We'll get on to postnatal recovery from diastasis recti in Chapter 9.

Now let's take a quick tour around the rest of our body, for a snapshot into what's going on elsewhere as we're growing our beautiful babies, before running through the best exercises to support a healthy pregnancy.

Hamstrings

The ripple effect of the prenatal tilted pelvis continues throughout the body, to surprising places like our hamstrings.

Hamstrings are the muscles that run down the back of our thighs. They attach to the bottom of our pelvis, on either side, and run from the sitz bones down the back of our leg to the back of our knee joints.

When people have achy hamstrings, it's often assumed that it's because they are tight and need to stretch, but actually, in pregnancy it can often be the opposite.

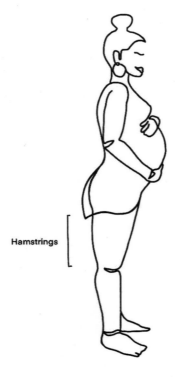

Hamstrings

The tilt in our pelvis and hollowing of our lower back can mean that our hamstrings are constantly held in an over-stretched position. This can be uncomfortable and for some may lead to sciatica-like pain. If you haven't yet heard of sciatica, count yourself fortunate because it's certainly not a barrel of laughs.

Sciatica is a pain often felt in the lower back and buttock, which is due to compression of the sciatic nerve. This nerve travels up the back of your leg, all the way from your foot to your lower back, via your hamstrings. If your hamstrings are overstretched, the sensations you're experiencing may be due to the neurological pain from this nerve, as opposed to the muscle itself.

In this case, the last thing we want is more stretching; what we actually need is to work on our posture, pelvic alignment and glute activation (strengthening our butt!).

I'd never experienced this before my twin pregnancy, but with the extra-large bump I felt it for the first time in my third trimester. Although the ache never completely went away, I found sitting down and working on a few pelvic tilt exercises for 5 minutes, twice a day, helped to alleviate some of the sensation. Postnatally, my symptoms eased quickly, within just a few weeks, but even now I remain aware of my posture when I lift, carry, feed and generally go about my daily mum-life activities.

So here are some of my favourite exercises for pregnancy fitness and core training, which will help to lay the foundation for a strong core in pregnancy, as well as glute activation moves and respiratory work (how we breathe).

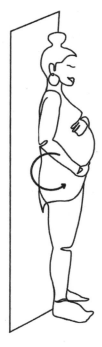

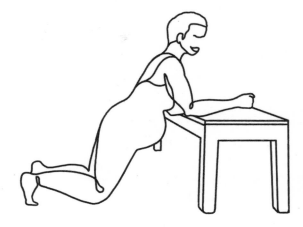

1

Standing pelvic tilt exercise

● Stand with your back against a flat wall, feet hip-width apart and 6 inches away from the wall. Inhale deeply and relax your back. Feel the relaxation through your spine.

● On your exhale, draw up your pelvic floor and press the small of your back against the wall, gently tilting your pelvis backwards. Hold this position for the duration of your exhale, about eight counts.

● Inhale and release.

● Repeat this exercise for a few minutes and then rest.

2

Modified planks (elevated)

● Kneel on the floor in front of a low, stable surface like a chair or bench.

● Place your forearms up onto the surface in front of you, bending both arms at the elbows.

● Sit up off your heels and take your knees back slightly so that you are able to shift your body weight forwards into a modified plank position, achieving a diagonal line from your neck all the way along your spine to your coccyx.

● Make sure that your hips are aligned and your glutes aren't pushing upwards.

● Hold this for 20–30 seconds before sitting back onto your heels and resting. Repeat for three sets if possible.

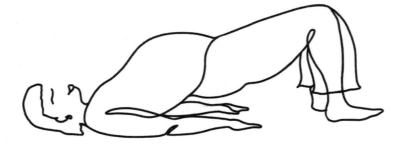

3

Bridge

Remember that performing exercises on your back for a short period of time is considered safe during pregnancy; however, if you feel uncomfortable or breathless in this position, cease the exercise immediately. In this case an exercise such as glute kickbacks (opposite) may be preferable.

● Lie flat on your back, with your arms by your sides, palms facing down. Bend both knees up so that the soles of your feet are flat on the floor. Keep your feet hip-width apart.

● Begin by inhaling through your nose. As you exhale, engage your glutes and lift your hips off the floor with control, until only your shoulders and feet are connected through the floor. Keeping your feet where they are, visualise drawing your heels further towards you to increase activation of your glutes.

● Hold for a count of four to eight and feel your glutes, back muscles and core working to hold this position.

● Return to the start position by slowly lowering your hips back towards the floor.

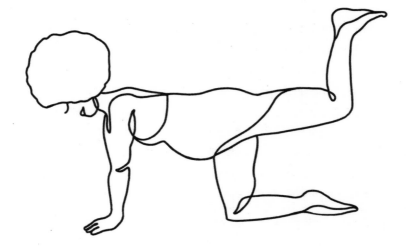

4

Glute kickbacks

● Start on all fours with your hands directly underneath your shoulders and your knees underneath your hips, hip-width apart.

● Keep your neck in optimal alignment by keeping your eyeline ahead on the floor in front of you. Avoid dropping your chin to your chest, or tilting your neck back by looking up too far.

● Lift one leg out behind you, keeping your knee bent at a 90-degree angle and keeping your heel flexed.

● The thigh of your raised leg should remain in line with your glutes and back. There should be no excessive arch in your lower back.

● Keeping the heel flexed, pulse the leg upwards by pushing the heel gently towards the ceiling. It's a small movement; your leg should only move a few centimetres up and down.

● Remember to keep good alignment from your neck along your spine to your glutes.

● Repeat this pulse for 30–40 seconds before lowering your knee back to the floor, returning to the start position.

● Rest and repeat on the other side.

A flexible floor

We can't talk about physicality in pregnancy without talking about how to train our pelvic floor in a little more detail.

All we seem to hear is how strong our pelvic floor needs to be during pregnancy, because of all the extra weight it's carrying. Whilst this is true, we should also give some attention to the need for a flexible floor as well. Labour would be an almost impossible task if all our pelvic floor did was hold on tight! This is a moment when relaxation is pivotal, so that our babies can descend down the birth canal and make their way out into the world. In fact, this is also why women might be told to relax their jaw during labour. As our jaw is connected to our core via the DFL (page 29), relaxation of the mouth can inspire relaxation down below.

I remember speaking at a fitness festival in my early twenties and being asked whether it's possible to overtrain your pelvic floor. I wish I could go back and answer that question again. I mumbled something about a 'well-rounded approach' to training your pelvic floor but, in all honesty, I hadn't yet fully grasped the true depth of its connection to the rest of the body. But let me tell you, it is possible to over-train your pelvic floor and finding the right balance of strength and relaxation is really important.

If we only ever contract this muscle group, we may develop an 'overactive' pelvic floor and begin to experience symptoms like difficulty urinating, painful sex, lower back ache and constipation. In this scenario Kegel exercises that encourage further tightening will only exacerbate the issue.

Relaxation of our pelvic floor should, in my opinion, be given just as much attention as strengthening. The following exercises are simple but may be a challenge if you're new to releasing the pelvic floor and rarely focus on letting go.

Pelvic floor relaxation exercise

● Rest back in a comfortable position, either propped up in bed or on the sofa with your arms and hands relaxed by your sides. If you're prenatal and don't feel comfortable resting back, you can sit on a chair with your feet placed hip-width apart, hands hanging loose by your sides or relaxed on your lap.

● Draw your attention on to your breath.

● With every inhale release the pelvic floor. You shouldn't feel as though you're bearing or pushing down, but rather you should feel a sensation of release.

● You may wish to place a hand on your belly to feel the rise and fall as you breathe. As you inhale and your stomach fills up, your pelvic floor should be relaxing.

● If possible, we can help to encourage pelvic floor relaxation by moving our legs into a frog position, with the soles of our feet together and knees bent, allowing them to fall out to the sides.

● If you are struggling to let go, visualisation can be a great help. As you inhale you want to imagine your vaginal muscles opening as well as your rear passage. You may wish to progress this by imagining a rose bud opening until you feel your pelvic floor soften.

● As you exhale, sigh out the breath through an open mouth. Don't try to tighten the pelvic floor on the exhale and instead focus solely on the release.

● Inhale and repeat.

● Remember this is not an active push or bearing down; this is about letting go.

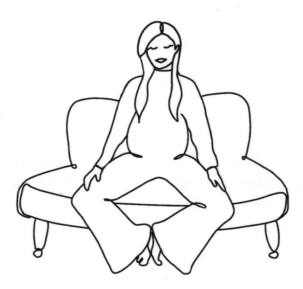

Glutes

There's another area that is prone to becoming extremely tight, causing extra tension for our deep core muscles, and that's our glutes. Although we know that weak glutes may be a contributor to sciatica-like pain, let's not confuse strong with over-tight. When a muscle is constantly in tension – and this goes for all muscles in the body – it cannot work properly. Tight glutes plague many of us. In fact, if I could draw your attention to your butt now and ask you to release, could you? Chances are you were actually clenching, without even knowing it.

Alongside stopping us from actually having strong and efficient muscles, tight glutes can pull our lower back and pelvis back out of alignment, actually in the exact reverse of the forwards pelvic tilt we mentioned which occurs naturally during pregnancy.

If you stand side on to a mirror and clench your bum tightly, you'll notice that as your butt tucks under, your pelvis is tilted backwards. Simultaneously your back will round and your shoulders hunch forwards. You might even find that you are now standing with your toes slightly turned out as overactive glutes can cause rotation at the hip joint, pushing your inner thighs forwards and out.

This rotation tracks down to our knees and feet, rotating them out also. A rotation like this can change how you stand and walk, and can even tug on the attachment ligaments to the pelvic floor, pulling them out of alignment too.

Wow! It just seems to go on and on, doesn't it? But, actually, it's simple: we just need to prioritise good posture and alignment.

If you think you might be a 'butt gripper' (I can barely type that with a straight face), I urge you to learn to let go!

A clue as to whether or not you are 'gripping' can be if you struggle to feel your glute muscles being activated at all. When muscles are over-tight, you won't feel them contracting, because they are already clenched. By relaxing them, stretching them or foam rolling, we can then begin to feel them engage again.

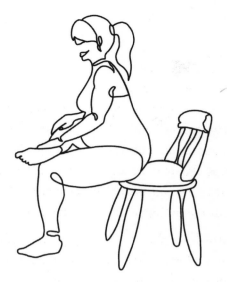

1

Seated glute stretch

This exercise is suitable for pre- and postnatal women, and helps us to release tension in our glutes and keeps our hips mobile without overstressing our joints.

● Sit on a chair with your feet flat on the floor, hip-width apart.

● Cross one leg over the other, so that one foot is resting on the knee of the supporting leg. It should look a little like the number 'four'.

● Inhale, and as you exhale slowly lean your chest forwards, maintaining a flat back until you feel the stretch in your lower back and buttocks.

● Visualise elongating the spine upwards and forwards as opposed to hunching over or curling the spine.

● Hold for 15–20 seconds.

● Inhale and gently return to the start position. Repeat.

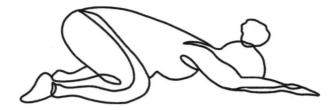

2

Child's pose

This exercise is great to encourage stretching of the hips, pelvis, lower back and thighs. It's suitable for pre- and postnatal women.

● Begin on all fours in the table-top position, with your knees placed directly under your hips.

● Create a V shape with your legs so that your big toes touch, unless you find this exerts too much pressure on your knees or doesn't allow enough room for your baby bump as you move into the next phase of the movement.

● Inhale and visualise your spine lengthening and elongating forwards.

● As you exhale take your butt towards your heels and lower your head towards the floor.

● Rest here with your forehead on the ground. If you find the floor too far away to rest your head comfortably, you may wish to use a folded blanket or yoga block to support your forehead.

● Extend your arms out fully in front of you.

● If you are postpartum and feel comfortable you may wish to sweep your arms backwards along your body, resting your hands, palms upwards, by your feet.

● Hold for 4–6 deep breaths. Return to the table-top position.

Note: *You want to avoid any pressure on your neck. If sweeping your arms back causes your body weight to shift onto your neck, return your arms to the forwards position or add a block as additional support under your forehead.*

3

Foam rolling

Foam rolling is a fantastic way to release tension in areas that might be tricky to target with stretching, such as our IT band, which runs along the outer length of our thigh. Foam rolling also helps us to increase circulation, which oxygenates the muscles. Below are three exercises that you can perform with a foam roller, during or after pregnancy.

As foam rolling is body weight compression, we need to be mindful of this at certain stages in pregnancy and in certain places along the body. You may wish to avoid engaging in deep-tissue manipulation and instead focus on light rolling to encourage circulation and relaxation.

There are also a few areas to avoid when working with a foam roller. We should never roll our joints, neck or lower back. There is also some evidence that some inner points of our calf muscle and adductor muscles (inner thigh) have been linked to inducing contractions, so, as a general rule of thumb, they, too, should be avoided.

Deeply rolling the underside of our feet should also be done with caution. There are some pressure points here that have been associated with stimulating the uterus enough to trigger labour. However, light rolling can be beneficial on the feet, especially if you have circulation issues.

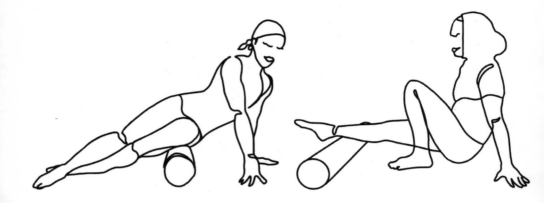

IT band

● Place your foam roller on the floor and sit on it, so that the length of your foam roller runs horizontally under your hips.

● Rotate onto your left hip, bringing your arms over the top of the roller, and place your palms on the floor.

● Your legs should be stacked on top of one another, with a slight bend at the knees, with your right foot relaxed on the floor just in front of your left, so that both feet are touching the floor.

● Use your feet to gently roll back and forth from your glute to the top of your thigh.

● Continue this for a few minutes, breathing evenly throughout. Then sit off the roller and relax before repeating on the other side.

Calves

● Sit on the floor with your legs stretched out in front of you. Bend your left leg up so that the sole of your left foot is on the floor.

● Place your foam roller horizontally underneath your right leg, just above your ankle, which is extended along the floor.

● Support yourself by placing both hands behind you on the floor.

● Use your hands and supporting left leg to lift your hips off the ground.

● Slowly move forwards and let the foam roller gently massage your right calf.

● Breathe evenly and continue rolling up and down for a few minutes.

● Lower your hips back to the floor and repeat on the other side.

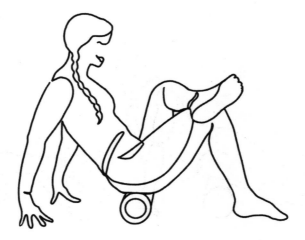

Glutes

● Start by placing your foam roller horizontally on the floor and lift yourself up to sit onto the roller so both glutes are resting on it.

● Place your hands on the floor behind you for support.

● Lift your left leg so that your left ankle rests onto your right leg, just below the knee. This will open up your hips.

● Rotate your body weight slightly to your left side to allow the change in body-weight pressure onto one side.

● Start gently rolling back and forth along the glute.

● Continue this for a few minutes, then rest both feet on the floor, resetting your body weight before repeating on the other side.

All of these exercises will help support a healthy and active pregnancy. Coming up, we look at which exercises are best suited to each stage of pregnancy and how our hormones change throughout the trimesters and can affect our fitness.

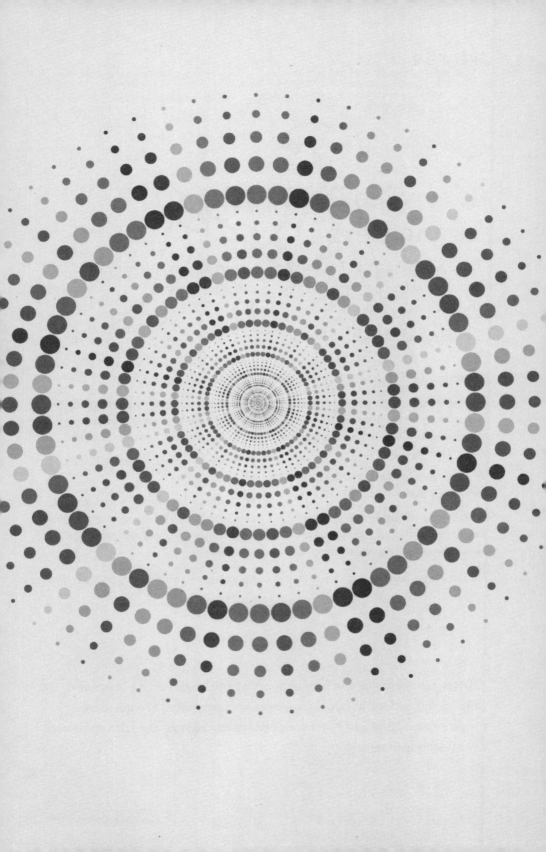

Exercise during the trimesters

Let's get down to the physical facts. Here are the recommendations for each trimester and some of my favourite exercises to support you along the way.

I want to make it clear right from the start that it's important you've been cleared to exercise by your medical team first. If you have any specific questions, don't hesitate to run them by your GP or midwife.

The following recommendations are pregnancy-specific and there are lots of progressions and modifications given. Enjoy!

The first trimester

Depending on how you're feeling in your first trimester, you might want to crawl under a blanket and just 'survive' the first few months of morning sickness or you might feel that you've got an extra bounce in your step.

Believe it or not, the first trimester has some great benefits for our fitness. In fact, the influence of early pregnancy on sporting performance is so impressive that it has even called into question whether this creates an uneven playing field for female athletes. During pregnancy, the amount of blood in our body increases, which is partly why we're so thirsty. Our body needs the increased water levels to meet the rising blood supply demand.

Higher levels of blood in our system mean that the amount of blood pumped around your body by a single heartbeat is increased too. This is known as 'stroke volume' and it increases steadily during the first two trimesters.

Our blood is responsible for carrying oxygen to our organs and muscles to help them function and recover. When we exercise, our muscles need more oxygen to have the energy to continue performing an activity. That's why our breathing becomes heavy and fast, as our body tries to meet the new oxygen demands by taking in more air.

Because of the natural increase in stroke volume during pregnancy (the amount of blood pumped by one heartbeat) a pregnant athlete will be transporting more oxygen throughout her body, without needing to raise her heart rate or breathe faster like non-pregnant women.

Stroke volume can rise between 20 and 100 per cent when you're pregnant compared to your pre-pregnancy levels. On average it rises by about 45 per cent, and for twin pregnancies about 15 per cent extra again.

I can remember so clearly that, before I'd had any type of scan in my first pregnancy, I felt an incredible rise in my energy levels (before the nausea came). I had always heard of pregnancy making you extra tired, so I was convinced we hadn't conceived. I just felt too good and that didn't match up with the stereotype of pregnancy I'd been told about. Once the pregnancy was confirmed I considered myself one of the 'lucky ones'. Blissfully unaware of the morning sickness that was waiting for me in just a few weeks, I revelled in this pregnancy feeling, with people even commenting on how upbeat and fresh-faced I looked. That 'pregnancy glow', I thought, which I now know is actually partly due to the increase in blood volume as it flushes our skin.

Stroke volume isn't the only increase we notice in early pregnancy that boosts our fitness ability. From the first trimester, a pregnant woman will also see a rise in red blood cell production. Red blood cells are responsible for carrying oxygen around our body. So, along with an increase in amount of blood in our body, during pregnancy our blood is like a super substance, with the higher red blood cell count meaning more oxygen is carried around our body at any time. This does, however, mean that we need more vitamins and iron to accommodate the raised levels of red blood cells. Gestational anaemia occurs if the body fails to meet these demands. If that happens, your midwife might prescribe you some iron supplements for the rest of the pregnancy.

Exercises for the first trimester

Generally speaking, the advice for the first trimester is that you can continue with your current exercise programme if you feel up to it – as long as your GP or midwife haven't indicated any reasons why it might be inadvisable.

For many women, though, pregnancy is the first time they've really given thought to working out, and in those cases it's important to build up slowly rather than jumping in at the deep end. It's great to get moving, and at times this can mean trying new things, especially if fitness in general is new to you, but now isn't the time to push extreme boundaries.

Jogging can be perfectly safe throughout pregnancy, provided you have experience running already. Try to pick routes with even surfaces as this limits the risk of falling. Also, and I'm speaking from personal experience here, it's a good idea to choose routes with easy access for a toilet break! I learned this the hard way in pregnancy number one!

There's not much you need to avoid in the first 3 months, but I would suggest staying clear of contact sports like boxing, kickboxing, judo or squash. You should also seek medical advice before continuing activities like horse riding or surfing where the risk of falling is increased.

Lots of ladies have questions about ab exercises in pregnancy. Generally, most abdominal movements are considered safe in the first trimester, but we should think about what's most beneficial, alongside what is safe.

We want to help our body prepare the best we can for a healthy pregnancy and labour. Crunches and sit-ups might be given the green light in the first 3 months of pregnancy, but that doesn't mean they're necessarily the best way to activate our core or prepare for pregnancy. There are so many other ways to train which can bring more advantages.

1
Travelling lunges

● Start standing with your feet hip-width apart. You need enough space to take about 10–20 steps forwards.

● Step forwards with your right foot.

● In this split-leg position lower your body so that both knees bend at a right angle. Your right thigh should now be parallel to the floor and your left thigh perpendicular to the floor.

● Push off your back foot, moving your body weight through the heel of your front foot to come to standing and join the back leg to your front.

● Step forwards with the left leg and repeat on the alternate side.

● Keep moving forwards in this way for 8 repetitions. Turn around and return to your starting position in the same way.

● For an extra challenge, extend your arms straight overhead and hold them here throughout this exercise.

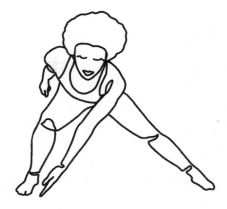

2
Side touches

● Begin standing with your feet hip-width apart and your arms relaxed by your sides.

● Inhale and step your right foot out to the side.

● Bend your right knee slightly, whilst reaching towards your right toe with your left hand.

● Keep your head up and back flat throughout. Let your right hand travel back a little, naturally.

● As you push off your right foot to return to the neutral start position, bring your arms back to your sides.

● Step immediately out with your left leg and repeat on the other side.

● Continue this sideways stepping motion for 20–40 seconds.

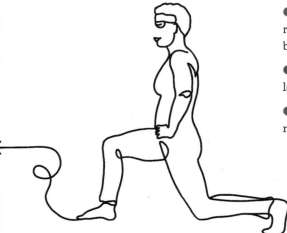

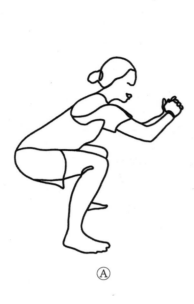

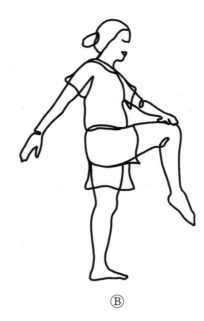

(A) (B)

3

Squat knee raises/kicks

● Stand with your feet slightly wider than hip-width apart and your hands relaxed by your sides.

● Inhale and bend your knees, sitting back into your hips until your thighs are parallel to the floor. Simultaneously bring your hands together in front of you with your arms slightly bent (image A).

● As you exhale push back up to standing and shift your weight onto one side, bringing the other knee up towards your chest (image B).

● Place the lifted foot back onto the floor and drop immediately back into a squat.

● Push up and shift onto the alternate side, bringing the other knee up to your chest.

● Continue to switch sides for the duration of the exercise, around 20–40 seconds.

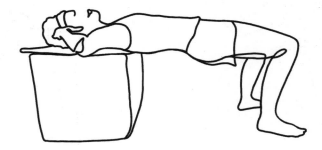

4

Hip thrusts

● Sit on the floor with your back against an exercise bench or a sofa, keeping your knees bent so that the soles of your feet are flat on the floor.

● Inhale and, as you exhale, begin this exercise by hinging your hips upwards so that your shoulders are now on the sofa and only your feet remain connected to the floor. You should be creating a line from your neck to your tailbone. Your knees should be bent to a 90-degree angle.

● Place your hands on top of your hip bones or behind your head for support but be careful not to tug your head out of alignment.

● Inhale and release your hips, lowering your pelvis back towards the floor.

● Immediately squeeze your glutes, exhale and lift your hips back up for the second rep of the exercise.

● Inhale and release your hips back to the start position. Repeat for 12–16 reps.

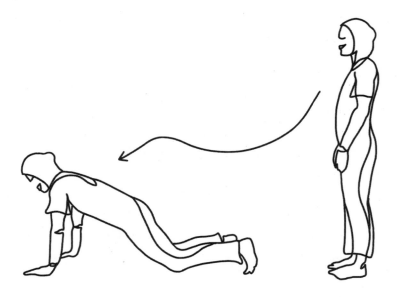

5

Modified inch worm

● Stand tall with your feet hip-width apart.

● Hinge forwards at the hips and walk your hands out in front of you along the floor, keeping your feet in place.

● As you walk your hands out in front of you, lower your knees to the floor until you have reached the half plank position.

● Hold this position for a few seconds before walking your hands backwards towards your feet, simultaneously lifting your knees back off the ground.

● Inhale and roll upwards to a standing position.

● Repeat for 8–10 reps.

Progression

● To progress this exercise, keep your knees off the ground as you walk your hands forwards and hold a full plank position.

● Try to keep your legs as straight as possible as you walk your hands back in, but bend if you need to.

● Inhale and roll back up to a standing position.

● Repeat for 8–10 reps.

These exercises don't need to be performed fast to be effective. It's all about technique.

How long you choose to perform each exercise will depend on your fitness level. On average you can aim for the recommended repetitions or try performing each exercise for 30–60 seconds. What's most important is that you always stay in tune with how you're feeling. We don't want to push ourselves to exhaustion, so exercising to a maximum of 80 per cent of our maximum effort at any given time is a good guideline. If you're unsure how to gauge this, there are certain body cues we can use to stay in touch with how our body is feeling. We'll go through these in more detail during the second trimester recommendations, but they can be useful even from this stage of pregnancy. If you feel dizzy, exhausted or notice any pain or excessive sweating, stop and rest. These can all be signs that you have pushed yourself towards exhaustion. If you notice any unusual bleeding or spotting, cease exercise and consult a medical professional.

Exercises for the second trimester

This is one of my favourite trimesters. Morning sickness fades (for most of us), and labour is still far enough away that we don't need to think about baby-proofing the house or broken-nights sleep just yet!

However, it is a time where we need to start adjusting our fitness programme again.

We've talked a lot about how pregnancy affects our core and lots of those changes really begin to take effect in the second trimester. My most frequently asked questions during this time are how much exercise is recommended and how long can you continue lifting weights. So, let's tackle those questions first!

How much exercise is safe?

When it comes to how much exercise you should be doing, it's probably one of those questions you've asked a thousand times only to encounter a frustrating answer that sounds something like 'it's different for each woman'. Whilst that is true, there is a little more we can add to the explanation that might help you find out what's the right amount of movement for you!

First up, I recommend working with exertion percentages, as opposed to timings. This means judging how an exercise feels and how much effort you're using, instead of how long you're doing it. I always advise my clients to work to approximately 60–70 per cent of their maximum exertion at any given time.[6]

I prefer working this way in pregnancy because it means we can always stay in touch with how our body is feeling in the moment. The intensity of exercise changes depending on how we feel at that time. Seventy per cent of our effort will be different from day to day depending on lots of factors, like our mood, whether we've had quality sleep or have any physical stresses. Even the position our baby is in in utero can impact how challenging a moment is. My twins twisted themselves into all sorts of interesting shapes. Anything but the textbook head down, by the end of it!

If you're looking for guidance on how many sessions you should do a week, and how long for, I'd suggest starting with 30–40 minutes of moderate-intensity exercise 3–5 days a week.

You may wish to increase this amount or duration, provided you have the time, but this should be checked with your GP or midwife first to get the all clear.

So what about weight training during pregnancy?

If you're interested in lifting weights, you might be feeling distinctly underwhelmed by the information that's out there on whether this is or isn't safe in pregnancy. It's not that there's a lot of conflicting information out there, it's just that there isn't really anything at all! The guidelines are vague, especially if you want to know specifics for each trimester.

If you like facts, according to a study released by the US National Library of Medicine, 'the adoption of a supervised, low-to-moderate-intensity strength-training programme during pregnancy can be safe and efficacious for pregnant women.'[7]

I told you. Very vague.

Personally, I always recommend functional training, which means training someone in a way to assist with everyday activities. For many women, this includes lifting and carrying. Suggesting that no pregnant woman lifts or carries for the entire gestational period is a little farfetched. Any pregnant woman who already has other children, for example, will know that motherhood isn't pausing for you while you put your feet up for 9 months. Car seats, highchairs and strollers all still need to be moved.

> **ANY PREGNANT WOMAN WHO ALREADY HAS OTHER CHILDREN, FOR EXAMPLE, WILL KNOW THAT MOTHERHOOD ISN'T PAUSING FOR YOU WHILE YOU PUT YOUR FEET UP FOR 9 MONTHS.**

During my third pregnancy, as a mum of two older children, I certainly had to do my fair share of hands-on parenting. There were plenty of times I had to lift my little ones into the bath or even protect them from hot lava by hoisting them onto a tower of safety cushions!

We can absolutely enjoy lifting weights throughout all trimesters, but we do want to make sure that we're not overloading our core or placing too much pressure on our joints. We should avoid lifting weights that are too heavy and only bring them overhead for a short period of time.

As for how much you can safely lift, we should aim for about 50–70 per cent of our pre-pregnancy maximum and this will be adjusted again come the third trimester.

If you're worried that you might push it a little too far, let me share some red flags which can indicate when a movement is too challenging.

Red flags

1 Technique is key. Our body is already undergoing a lot of changes during pregnancy and we don't want to add undue pressure onto already stressed joints. **Arching too much in the lower back, clenching your jaw** or **curling your toes** in order to perform a movement are all signs that an exercise is too challenging at this time. We can work up to it, but if you notice any of these signs, take a step back and build up slowly and with correct technique.

2 We also want to stay aware of our body temperature. Naturally our core temperature is higher when we're pregnant, and our body temperature will rise when we're exercising too, but **profuse sweating** or **feeling overheated** or **dizzy** is another sign that a movement is too strenuous and we should look to reduce the intensity.

3 Any **pain in the back or pelvis** is also a sign that we may be overdoing it. With pregnancy hormones playing a role in loosening our ligaments we want to make sure that we aren't over-stretching or straining during movement. For any women who develop pelvic girdle pain (page 108), wide stances such as sumo squats or lateral lunges may need to be avoided.

4 Any **spotting or bleeding** is cause to cease exercise and check in with your medical team. There's no need to panic – spotting in early pregnancy can be completely natural – but it's best to get in touch with your GP and midwife if you have any concerns.

5 Noticing **an increase in Braxton Hicks contractions** is also something to be mindful of. This isn't necessarily a reason to avoid exercise completely, but you might want to adjust movements and reduce the intensity accordingly.

Reducing intensity

As pregnancy progresses and we start to really feel the effects of our growing bump and fluctuating hormones, we can still enjoy exercise but we should reduce its intensity.

Intensity is how hard we're working at any given time. Taking intensity down doesn't mean we won't be getting a good workout in. There are a few ways we can adapt our exercise but still reap the benefits.

Using levels is one of my favourite ways to either increase or decrease the intensity of a movement, and it's accessible for everyone. Take a chair, bench or step, for example. These are all great ways to reduce or, when you're ready, up intensity.

A half plank is a good example. As I moved through my twin pregnancy I began to feel that the all-fours position felt uncomfortable on the front of my abdomen. The increased weight of the babies was creating too much pressure, so to reduce this I simply took my palms off the floor and placed them onto a seat or step bench. By lifting my upper body up in this way, I created a diagonal line from my head to my tailbone, meaning that the load placed onto my core was reduced. We can use this position for lots of exercises like press-ups, modified burpees or the cat-cow stretch.

Of course, we always want to make sure that any level we're using, such as a chair or step, is solid, safe and won't move or slip.

Towards the later stages of the second trimester we might also want to consider reducing the impact in our movements.

Impact refers to any movement when we come into forcible contact with the ground when we land. We can reduce impact easily, by taking out any jumps, hops or skips. A lunge hop, for example, becomes a straight lunge with a knee raise, keeping the supporting leg on the ground (demonstrated in exercise 1). Another example would be adapting something like the traditional burpee (I feel exhausted just writing the word). Instead of the jump we can opt for a straight arm reach or a step up. This still requires energy and cardio fitness, but we've removed the impact, reducing the risk of injury.

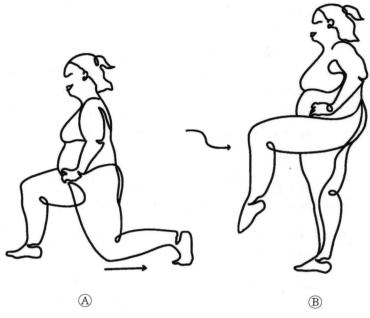

1

Reverse lunge with knee raise

● Begin standing tall with your feet hip-width apart, arms relaxed by your sides.

● Inhale and take a step back with your left foot.

● Bend both knees to 90-degree angles, so that your back knee hovers just off the floor (image A).

● As you exhale push back up to your split stance standing position, transferring your weight onto your front, right leg.

● Immediately lift your left foot up off the floor and bring your left knee towards your chest (image B).

● Inhale and place your left foot back on the floor behind you to prepare for the second rep.

● Repeat 8–10 reps on the same side. After the final rep bring your left foot back in line with your right foot, hip-width apart in a neutral stance.

● Repeat on the other side.

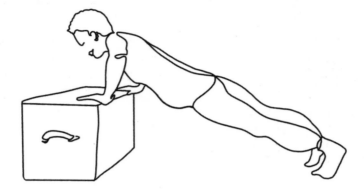

2

Elevated press-ups

● Stand facing a bench or other supportive elevated platform.

● Place your hands onto the bench, just wider than shoulder-width apart.

● Walk your feet back so that your body reaches a full plank position, until you create a diagonal line along your spine from your neck to your tailbone.

● When you're ready, inhale and bend your elbows, so that your chest lowers towards the bench. Keep your body straight throughout this movement.

● Exhale and push away from the bench until your elbows are extended but not locked.

● Inhale and repeat for 8–10 repetitions.

Modification

Note: the higher the platform, the more the intensity will reduce for your core. For beginners this exercise can also be performed on your knees.

3

Modified burpees

● Stand facing a bench, chair or other supported platform.

● Inhale and bend your knees, placing your hands onto the platform in front of you (image A).

● Take your left leg straight out and place it on the floor behind you so that it is fully extended. Immediately bring your right foot back in line with your left, keeping them hip-width apart (image B).

● As you exhale reverse this motion by stepping back in, first with your left and then with your right foot. You should now be back in the squat position with feet hip-width apart.

● Push up to standing and reach your arms up overhead.

● Inhale and repeat this motion for 10–12 reps.

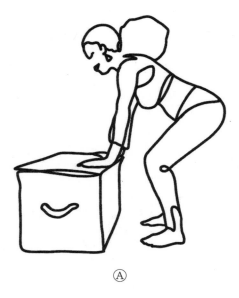

Ⓐ

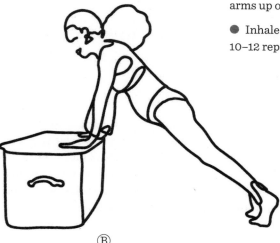

Ⓑ

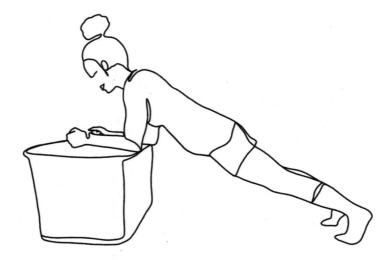

4

Modified plank

● Place both of your elbows onto a bench, chair or other supported platform.

● Inhale and walk your feet back so that your body reaches a plank position. You should be in a diagonal line, keeping your spine in good alignment from your neck to your tailbone.

● With each exhale gently draw up your pelvic floor and deep core muscles.

● Hold this position for 15–30 seconds, breathing in and out continually.

● Walk your feet back in or gently lower your knees onto the floor to relax.

● Repeat for 2–3 reps if you feel up to it.

Modification

To modify this exercise and reduce the intensity, keep your knees on the floor throughout, shifting the majority of your body weight forwards onto your arms so you are in a half plank position, with a diagonal line from your neck to your tailbone.

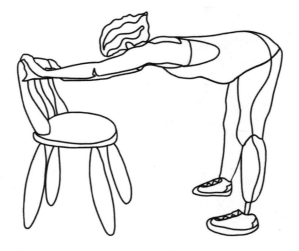

5

Back and hamstring stretch using chair

● Stand in front of a high platform such as a sideboard, work surface or the back support of a chair.

● Place your hands onto the support.

● Inhale and walk your feet backwards a few paces. Shoot your hips backwards, so that you hinge forwards at the hips, creating a 90-degree angle at your waist, so that your chest is parallel to the floor and your legs are straight but not locked.

● In this position shift your weight from side to side, moving your hips gently from left to right. Feel the stretch down the back of your legs and sides of your back as you move.

● After 10–20 seconds slowly walk your feet back in and return to standing.

The third trimester

In this final trimester the focus shifts to labour preparation. Pelvic floor work, both strengthening and relaxation, becomes even more of a priority. We also want to prepare all our core stabiliser muscles (glutes, TVA, back muscles and leg muscles) to help with an active and mobile labour.

We still want to reduce any impact or perhaps take it out completely, depending on how we're feeling. If in any doubt, speak to your medical team for advice; however, the best exercises I would recommend are all those to get your body prepared for the big day!

Labour preparation exercises

An active and mobile labour is when the mother chooses to move around the room and adopt different positions, based on natural instincts, to facilitate the birthing process. Whether you choose to birth this way, or just use these exercises for the early stages of labour, they are still great to get your body ready for birth.

Active birth positions may include full squats, hovering, four-point kneeling position, crouching, pushing, pulling or squeezing. That's a lot of work for our body, so let's use pregnancy to help it build strength to prepare.

First, here are the answers to the questions I'm asked most frequently on third trimester training.

Can you lie on your back?

I'm asked this a lot by clients at this stage of pregnancy. The truth is that there's a difference between lying on your back in general and lying on your back to perform an exercise, and these things should be treated differently.

Once you reach 16–20 weeks pregnant, your uterus is large enough that when lying on your back, in supine (flat out) or semi-supine (knees bent), you can place too much pressure on the vena cava.

Your vena cava is a large blood vessel running along the posterior (back) of the abdominal wall. If this blood vessel becomes compressed, it could restrict blood flow, and make you feel dizzy, nauseous or faint. In extreme cases of prolonged compression this could potentially restrict blood flow to yourself and baby.

However, although this sounds like an instant red flag and something to avoid completely, the guidance is that you *can* perform exercises on your back for a short amount of time but only if you feel comfortable. Using the previous red flags can indicate whether you should continue to exercise on your back or avoid this position until after delivery.

Personally, I felt confident performing exercises on my back during both my singleton pregnancies, but one day in the third trimester with the twins, I rolled onto my back when lying in the garden and felt dizzy almost instantly. I decided to stop exercising on my back at this point, and instead would lie sideways or exercise sitting on a chair.

Here's my go-to third trimester circuit!

IN THIS FINAL TRIMESTER THE FOCUS SHIFTS TO LABOUR PREPARATION. PELVIC FLOOR WORK, BOTH STRENGTHENING AND RELAXATION, BECOMES EVEN MORE OF A PRIORITY.

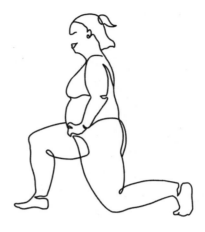

1

Forward lunge

● Stand with your feet hip-width apart, hands on your hips.

● Inhale and take a wide step forwards with your left foot.

● Bend both knees to a 90-degree angle, so that your right knee hovers just off the floor.

● Exhale and push off the front foot to return to a neutral stance position.

● To progress this exercise, lift your arms straight up overhead as you step forwards and hold them above your head as you bend into the full lunge and return to standing.

● Repeat for 8–10 reps.

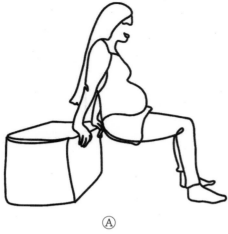

(A)

2

Tricep dips from a chair

● Sit on a chair and grip the edges of the seat either side of your hips, so that your fingers are pointed at the floor.

● Walk your feet a few paces forwards and press your palms into the seat, so that your hips lift off the seat and move slightly in front of the chair. You should now be supporting your weight with your hands (image A).

● Keep your knees bent and the soles of your feet flat to the floor.

● Bend your elbows to between a 45- and 90-degree angle and lower your hips towards the floor (image B).

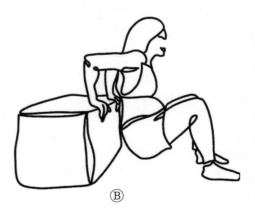

(B)

● Push back up through your palms, straightening your arms but not locking them.

● Continue this up-and-down motion for 6–10 reps.

● After the final rep, shift your hips backwards, sitting back onto the chair and relaxing your arms by your sides.

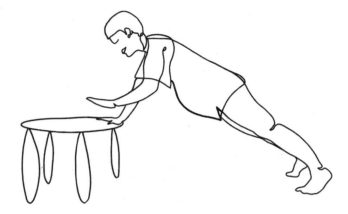

3

Modified plank (elevated) with arm raise

This exercise activates the deep core muscles and encourages stability of the pelvis.

● Place your palms onto a bench, chair or other supported platform.

● Walk your feet back so that your body reaches a full plank position, until you create a diagonal line from your neck to your tailbone.

● You may choose to hold this position for the full duration of the exercise.

Progression

● If you'd like to *progress* this, you may wish to begin marching your arms by gently lifting your hands off the platform one at a time.

Modification

● To modify this exercise and reduce the intensity, lower your knees down to the ground so you are in an elevated half plank position.

● First reach forwards with your left hand, extending your left arm so that your arm reaches in line with your ear.

● Place your left hand back onto the platform and repeat with your right.

● Continue alternating arm raises for 8–10 reps and hold the exercise for the remainder of the hold.

● Hold for 20–30 seconds.

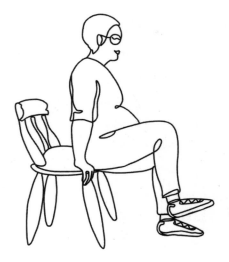

4

Seated, single-leg lift core exercise (pelvic floor)

● Sit on the edge of a chair, with your back straight and your shoulders back. Lift up so that your spine maintains good alignment and all three natural curves are present at the neck, thorax and lumbar spine. (See page 170.)

● Take a few deep breaths in this position.

● Inhale, and as you exhale, draw up your pelvic floor and deep core muscles by visualising your coccyx and pubic bone coming together and lifting up.

● As you do this, gently lift your left leg a few centimetres off the floor, keeping your knee bent and foot flexed.

● Inhale and release your leg back to the floor. Repeat on the other side.

● Continue this for 6 reps each side.

Mobility circuit

As we move through the third trimester, we can begin to reduce our exertion percentage down to 50 per cent, or lower if we feel it's necessary.

If you feel like you might be ready to reduce any structured workouts and instead would prefer some gentle mobility actions to keep joints moving and muscles relaxed, here are a few exercises that might be just right.

I started these types of workouts around 32 weeks when pregnant with my twins, and about 35 weeks with my singleton pregnancies.

1

Mini squats with arm swings

● Stand tall with your arms relaxed by your sides and your feet hip-width apart.

● Inhale and relax your knees so that they bend very slightly.

● Exhale and push through your heels to straighten your legs, without locking them.

● Simultaneously swing your arms out to the sides and overhead, so that they meet just above your head.

● Inhale and bend your knees slightly, letting your arms relax back down to your sides.

● Repeat these gentle swings for 20 seconds.

2

Supported leg swings

● Stand side on, with your left side next to a sideboard or the back of a chair or bench.

● Place your left hand onto the sideboard for support.

● Inhale and take your left leg slightly out behind you, balancing gently on one leg, holding on to the sideboard.

● Exhale and let your left leg relax and swing forwards.

● Continue this swinging motion whilst breathing in and out regularly.

3

Ankle rolls

● Sit on the edge of a chair, with your back straight and your shoulders back.

● Gently lift one foot off the floor and roll your ankle around in circles, by drawing a circle in the air with your toes.

● Perform 8–10 rolls to the left and 8–10 rolls to the right.

● Repeat on the other side.

5

Elevated 'good toes naughty toes'

● Sit on the floor or a chair and raise your feet up onto a platform like a chair, bench or sofa. Place your hands on the ground behind you for support.

● Breathe in and out deeply, and as you do so point and flex your toes alternately.

● Continue for 10–16 reps each side.

4

Sit to standing with foot march

● Sit on the edge of a chair, with your back straight and your shoulders relaxed.

● Inhale and, as you exhale, push through both feet and come to a standing position.

● Once you reach standing, immediately march on the spot, bringing your knees towards your bump, first lifting one foot and then the other. Inhale and return to a seated position.

● Continue this motion for 8–10 reps.

Perineal massage

Finally, when talking about labour preparation, we should mention a very important part of our anatomy, the perineum.

If you hadn't heard of this word before reading this book, don't worry; you are not alone. Although we've seen a big improvement in pelvic health awareness over the last few years, many women still aren't aware of exactly how their pelvic floor muscles look or where they're located. Giving birth without understanding your pelvic floor structure is like getting on a horse without knowing how to ride: doable, but reckless. So, let's figure things out together now.

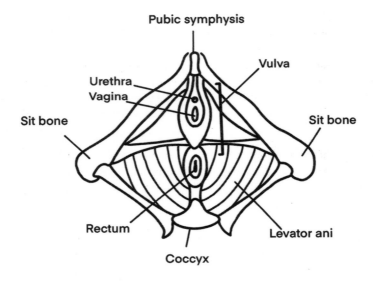

The perineum is a muscle that lies just in front of the rest of your pelvic floor sling. It's the technical term for the muscle and skin between your vagina and rectum. This stretches significantly during vaginal delivery. At the end of the third trimester we can begin perineal massage to help prepare this area for dilation and crowning by gently massaging and stretching the perineal tissues. This has many benefits including reducing the risk of a tear or need for an episiotomy, reducing perineal pain and reducing the length of the second stage of labour.

My close friend and women's health physiotherapist Clare Bourne (@clarebournephysio) kindly lent her expertise to this chapter, offering her best advice on how to begin perineal massage during pregnancy.

'We can begin perineal massage any time after 35 weeks,' Clare told me. 'We recommend it to women as research has shown that this can significantly reduce the risk of tearing during delivery. Not all women find it easy to do, or feel comfortable with it, but it is important that we're all educated about it and feel empowered to give it a go.'

Perineal massage exercise

To do perineal massage we need to find a relaxed position, for example sitting propped up in bed; if, however, you find it difficult to reach around your bump, you may find it easier to place one foot up on the toilet seat. Below is a step-by-step guide to help you start perineal massage:

● Wash your hands and apply a natural lubricant to the vulva, vaginal opening and your thumb.

● Place your thumb approximately one inch inside the vagina and gently sweep side to side 10 times. Think about the area like a clock, with 12 o'clock at the top near the pubic bone and 6 o'clock at the coccyx. You are aiming to sweep between 3 and 9 o'clock. You should feel a stretch but it shouldn't be painful.

● Next, gently stretch in each direction from 3 to 9 o'clock and hold each stretch for 20–30 seconds.

● Aim to do this 1–2 times a week until delivery.

Please note: *Do not do perineal massage if you have vaginal bleeding, an active infection or any rupture of membranes.*

Mind towards motherhood

Exercising in the run-up to labour is a great way to help our bodies prepare for the big day. However, it's not just physical preparation that we need.

My good friend, Siobhan Miller (@shivy_miller), who is a licensed hypnobirthing instructor, was instrumental in preparing me mentally for my second and third births. Founder of The Positive Birth Company, Siobhan has dedicated her career to helping women prepare for birth by inviting calming thoughts and positivity.

'Doing what you can to prepare both physically and mentally for labour and ensure a positive birth experience is 100 per cent worth it,' Siobhan told me when we first met. 'Because your birth experience is not just one day; it's something you carry with you forever.

'If your birth is a positive and empowering experience, you will carry this memory and confidence with you throughout motherhood. Every time you recall your birth you will be reminded of how strong, capable and powerful you really are. You cannot put a value on this! It's like having a superpower you can tap into any time you need.

'On the other hand, if you feel like you're out of control and panicked giving birth, this is what you will remember. Your risk of suffering from postnatal anxiety or depression is increased and you may even experience post-traumatic stress disorder (PTSD). Anxiety, depression and PTSD can impact all areas of your life from your wellbeing to bonding with your baby, to other relationships you have.'

Knowing Siobhan on a personal level, I'm aware that she speaks not just as a professional but also as a mother, having experienced the value of a healthy mindset during her own deliveries.

'Throughout my second labour I felt calm, confident and in control. I was listened to, respected and well supported. Things weren't completely straightforward but I felt confident, capable and invincible. The polar opposite to how I felt after my first son was born,' Siobhan told me.

I had actually met Siobhan for the first time during my second pregnancy, and as I was adamant I wanted another epidural, I thought hypnobirthing wouldn't apply to me. Isn't it just for women opting for a home birth or birthing pool, I thought? But Siobhan made it clear: hypnobirthing can be useful for *all* women!

'No matter how you choose to give birth, having a positive connection between your body and mind can be instrumental to feeling calm and in control during your labour.'

I later found out just how true this was, particularly after I was booked in for a caesarean section with my twins. Heading into the unknown, with my first twin pregnancy, not to mention during a global pandemic, and all whilst moving house and homeschooling for the first time, I began to teeter on the edge of feeling overwhelmed. But thanks to my use of breathing practices, mantras and relaxation techniques, I actually found my twin birth an incredibly powerful, positive and calming birth experience.

NO MATTER HOW YOU CHOOSE TO GIVE BIRTH, HAVING A POSITIVE CONNECTION BETWEEN YOUR BODY AND MIND CAN BE INSTRUMENTAL TO FEELING CALM AND IN CONTROL DURING YOUR LABOUR.

Mantras for a better birth

I asked Siobhan to share a few of her favourite mantras, for any prenatal ladies who might want to give this a go:

1 '"My surges cannot be stronger than me, because they are me",' Siobhan told me. 'This is so true and hopefully reassuring. It reminds us that nothing is happening *to* us; *we* are doing it!'

2 '"Every surge brings me closer to meeting my baby" is another favourite,' Siobhan said. 'I like this because it's a good reminder that labour is a positive pathway to meeting our baby. We can all sometimes lose sight of this, and this is a fab reminder.'

3 'Finally I love "Birth is powerful, but so am I". It's such a positive and empowering statement. However we birth our babies, the fact that we have grown an entire human and brought new life into the world is nothing short of miraculous!'

I felt empowered just listening to Siobhan speak so passionately about these mantras and her advice didn't stop there. 'Mantras are just one way to prepare for our labour,' Siobhan told me. 'I teach people to use all five of their senses as a checklist to transform their environment into one that is calm, relaxing, familiar and more conducive for birth as well.'

WHEN YOU'RE GIVING BIRTH YOU WANT TO FEEL RELAXED AND UNINHIBITED, SO PACK ITEMS IN YOUR BIRTH BAG THAT WILL ENABLE YOU TO MEET EACH ONE OF YOUR SENSES WITH SOMETHING THAT AIDS RELAXATION AND MAKES YOU FEEL GOOD.

Birth with your senses

'We subconsciously "read" the world around us through our senses,' Siobhan shared. 'And this informs how we feel in any given space. If a room smells nice and looks nice (think of a spa), you immediately feel more relaxed in it. If you enter a room which smells unpleasant, doesn't appear very comfortable and you can hear lots of noise, you will probably feel more on edge. When you're giving birth you want to feel relaxed and uninhibited, so pack items in your birth bag that will enable you to meet each one of your senses with something that aids relaxation and makes you feel good.

'For example, you could pack a string of fairy lights or battery-operated tea lights; you could pack an eye mask; you could pack a diffuser for essential oils or a room spray; you might make a playlist and pack headphones or a bluetooth speaker; you could pack your favourite energy-boosting snacks and drinks and, finally, things that feel comforting and familiar to touch – maybe a pillow or cushion from home or a blanket or throw.

'Simply by using this collection of items, in just a matter of minutes, you have the power to transform even a very clinical setting into a space that is lit by fairy lights, smells like a spa with happy music playing and you can rest on a blanket from home whilst eating your favourite snacks! Bliss!'

It occurred to me, as I wrote out the notes from this conversation, that this all sounded pretty relaxing even now, although I'm not heading into labour. As I write, I'm perched on the edge of my bed, the rest of which is covered in a mountain of washing. The children have gone to sleep and the above is sounding very tempting. I feel as though now might be a great time to take some of my advice (or Siobhan's to be more accurate) and set up a relaxing environment with my favourite music and snacks and have myself a relaxing bath. I'll be right back in the next chapter with an insight into how our hormones change during pregnancy and the effect it can have on our fitness.

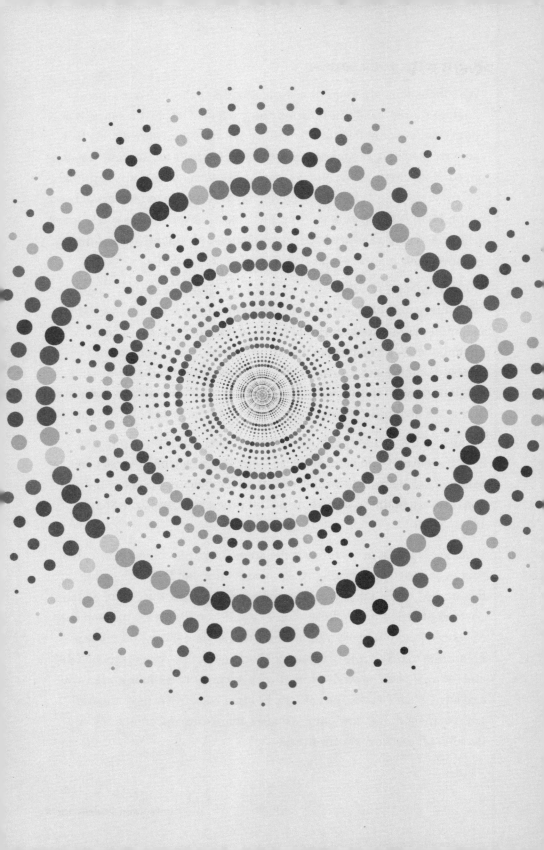

Pregnancy hormones

Ah, hormones, those lovely little things that have my husband running for cover once a month. In this chapter we look at the changes in our hormone levels during pregnancy and how they can affect our exercise programme.

I'll admit, I'm not the most upbeat pregnant person. I certainly didn't skip through the trimesters, and don't get me started on morning sickness. Which, incidentally, is a horrible example of false advertising. It is *not* isolated to the mornings like the name suggests. Well, not for me at least, and according to research not for between 50 and 60 per cent of other women either.[8]

The hormone believed to be responsible for morning sickness is called human chorionic gonadotropin (hCG) and it's also this hormone which is most commonly used to detect a pregnancy using a home pregnancy kit.

hCG

If I'm honest, I have mixed emotions about this hormone. As soon as I saw the line fade up on the pregnancy test, which confirmed my second pregnancy, I felt its presence looming, because although I was ecstatic about the pregnancy, I also knew what the effects of this hormone could mean.

My experience with morning sickness in the past is that it's one of the few times I have felt out of control of my body. Other women seem to sail through the first trimester, either not feeling sick at all, or just handling it much better than I could.

You know when you're younger and told that once you throw up on a spirit, you'll never want to drink it again? That's sort of how I feel about everything that got me through morning sickness. From the podcasts I listened to to distract myself, to the fizzy water I sipped daily or the over-consumption of breaded chicken, which was the only food to stay down. All of it is now solidly a 'no-go' area!

However, despite giving us the 'ick', the actual purpose of hCG is fascinating and important.

Produced within the first 2 weeks after conception, once the embryo implants into our uterus, hCG encourages our body to continue producing the hormone progesterone. Progesterone prevents menstruation, thereby providing protection for the uterus lining and our pregnancy.

Truth be told, the link between morning sickness and hCG is still the subject of research. But one idea is that nausea is the body's reaction to the rapid rise in hCG, which reaches its peak towards the end of the first trimester.

Despite this uncomfortable side effect, prenatal nausea is actually a way of our body protecting both mother and baby. It's thought that morning sickness helps our body to recognise foods that might contain harmful toxins. That's not to say that those who don't experience it are in danger; many find they feel bright throughout all the trimesters, and even those of us who do have nausea will experience varying degrees.

So why is hCG relevant for pregnancy fitness?

If you do find that you're feeling a little green in those first few weeks, exercise might be the furthest thing from your mind. In all of my pregnancies I barely poked my head over the duvet between weeks 6 and 16. When I could manage it, though, a short walk around the block or sitting outside in a chair to breathe some fresh air did wonders to lift my mood and relax my body. However, I'm a huge supporter of listening to your body and if it's your mattress rather than the exercise mat you're craving, go with your instincts!

hCG levels drop back to pre-pregnancy levels at around 3 weeks after giving birth. This sudden drop can leave some women feeling down or suffering with symptoms of depression.[9] How we feel emotionally greatly impacts how we feel physically, so although industry guidelines say that, 'provided there are no medical complications, women can begin pelvic floor exercises and walks immediately after birth,' that doesn't mean you'll feel ready to. Our mood and mental wellbeing dictates how we cope with physical changes and we have to make sure we feel ready to exercise before we get started.

hCG is just one of the hormones impacting us physically during pregnancy. There are many more at play that we need to be aware of.

So let's have a look at the head honchos, progesterone and oestrogen. We simply can't discuss pre- and postnatal life without them!

Oestrogen

Incredibly, research has found that a woman will produce more oestrogen during one pregnancy than throughout her entire life when not pregnant.[10]

That blew my mind when I first read it. It gives us an inkling into the huge amounts of hormones fluctuating through our bodies during the trimesters.

Oestrogen enables our uterus to grow. It also helps us maintain the uterine lining, supports the development of our baby's organs and regulates levels of other hormones in our body. Later on in pregnancy, the presence of oestrogen helps to prepare our breasts for breastfeeding, by enlarging the nipples and encouraging milk gland development.

INCREDIBLY, RESEARCH HAS FOUND THAT A WOMAN WILL PRODUCE MORE OESTROGEN DURING ONE PREGNANCY THAN THROUGHOUT HER ENTIRE LIFE WHEN NOT PREGNANT.

So why is this relevant to pregnancy exercise?

Oestrogen itself doesn't have a direct impact on our exercise programme, but the changes it inspires in our body does. Breast enlargement, for example, can alter how we sit or stand. The weight of our increased breast size can change our posture by rounding our shoulders forwards, causing our upper back muscles to become over-stretched, whilst the chest muscles become tight. For this reason we want to work on exercises that can help us manage our posture and also stretch across the chest to release any building tension.

Progesterone

The next big player, progesterone, starts affecting our body even before conception. During our menstrual cycle it helps to thicken the lining of our uterus in preparation for implantation of a fertile egg.

As our pregnancy progresses, progesterone levels in our body continue rising. One effect of this hormone is that it relaxes the smooth muscles in our uterus, bladder, bowel and veins. The smooth muscle in the uterus is relaxed to help prevent contractions early on in pregnancy. But, as the smooth muscle in the bowel is also relaxed, our digestive process can be affected. Contraction of this area plays a big part in ensuring regular bowel motions, so it's not uncommon for women to sometimes experience constipation in pregnancy.

Progesterone's main role is to help us sustain and develop our pregnancy. As if that wasn't already a full-time job, progesterone also encourages the production of breastmilk and dilates our blood vessels.

Finally, progesterone is thought to suppress the production of an enzyme in the brain called monoamine oxidase (MAO). MAO has been linked with depression, which many people believe is why you may feel euphoric during pregnancy. Immediately after childbirth, however, levels of progesterone drop quickly, which throws MAO levels out of balance, potentially contributing to the 'baby blues' and feelings of depression or overwhelm postpartum.

Why is this important for pregnancy exercise?

Another byproduct of progesterone is that it increases our body temperature, meaning you'll naturally be feeling warmer during pregnancy. If we add exercise into the mix, it becomes even more important to stay hydrated and increase our fluid intake. Any time we feel dizzy, drained or as though we're overheating, it's important to rest and take a break.

Serotonin

Serotonin doesn't get nearly as much attention as it should. I found it fascinating when I first started learning about its role, and it changed a lot about how I moved through my pregnancies.

The impact of serotonin can be relevant whether you are prenatal, postnatal or consider yourself neither. Largely produced in our gut, serotonin is known as a 'happy hormone', along with endorphins, which you might have heard of.

When we take a deep breath in, our body can utilise the action of the descending diaphragm to massage our intestines, which stimulates the production of serotonin and boosts happy feelings.

Why is this important for pregnancy exercise?

Well, despite being produced mostly in the gut, serotonin is released all along the spinal cord and throughout our brain. It's known for its effect on our mood and can be a great tool when we need an energy boost or want to feel positive and relaxed. Exercises like three-dimensional breathing (page 39) or mindfulness practices such as the body scan (page 31) are both fab to encourage serotonin production.

There is also a small amount of research that has suggested that serotonin promotes muscle growth. So far this research has only been tested 'in vitro' (which means, in a glass, in a laboratory test site) so we'll have to reserve judgement but it will be interesting to see how the research progresses.[11]

Relaxin

The clue is in the name on this one!

The hormone relaxin's main function is to loosen, or 'relax', the ligaments around our pelvis in preparation for labour. This 'loosening' of our joints means that our pelvis can be more mobile for delivery and the baby can descend smoothly down the birth canal. Relaxin will also help to soften and widen our cervix during birth.

Relaxin is produced as early as 2 weeks after conception and can stay in our system for up to 5 months postpartum or longer if you choose to breastfeed.

Although this loosening effect is aimed at getting our pelvic area ready for labour, we can't isolate the effect to just one part of our body. All our joints will be affected, meaning they are less stable than before.

How does relaxin affect pregnancy exercise?

When we're exercising in pregnancy, we should be aware of this change to our joints and ligaments and make sure that we don't overstretch or overload any joints that are already compromised by the loosening effects of relaxin. This is why I recommend dropping your weight-lifting maximum to 50–70% as pregnancy goes on. The effects of relaxin can sometimes be so strong that it is often thought of as a main contributor to pelvic girdle pain (PGP) or symphysis pubis dysfunction (SPD).

If you're wondering what PGP or SPD are, then chances are you most likely haven't experienced them, or at least not to a high level. For those that do experience them, there is a wide scale of how intense symptoms might be.

Pelvic girdle pain and SPD

SPD and PGP are often used to describe the same thing, but there is a difference.

Symphysis pubis dysfunction (SPD) is the name for when pain is felt specifically at the front of the pelvis, where the symphysis pubic joint is positioned.

Pain can be caused if the joint begins to move unevenly during pregnancy, due to an imbalance in the core. The baby's weight and position can also contribute to sensations of SPD as it places pressure on our pelvis.

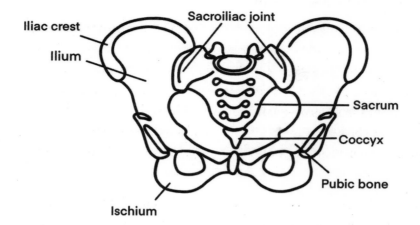

Pelvic girdle pain (PGP), on the other hand, is the term used to describe pain or discomfort in all other areas of the pelvis, such as at the rear, by the coccyx; at the sides of the pelvis; or underneath. In recent years, pelvic girdle pain has become the more commonly used term to describe all pelvic pain in pregnancy.

PGP has many other nicknames, such as 'lightning crotch' or 'groin pain'. It can be incredibly uncomfortable but there are no harmful effects to mum or baby. Up to 45 per cent of women experience this during the prenatal period and up to 25 per cent will feel its effects postpartum.

Although relaxin has been viewed as one of the main causes of PGP, there are other contributing factors too, such as changes in posture during pregnancy, the increased weight of the uterus and the position of the baby. It's also thought that emotional stress can cause aches in this area and affect our body's ability to recover.

Why is relaxin important for prenatal exercise?

Because of the effect this hormone has on our joints, we need to make some adaptations to how we exercise. We want to stay aware of how it feels when we perform movements that require wide-legged stances, as they could increase the strain on our joints. If your pelvis is aching, bending into a deep squat isn't going to help ease the pain or support recovery. Alongside avoiding over-stretching joints that are already suffering, we should also be mindful of single-sided exercises, like standing on one leg or running. A pelvis managing PGP needs equal balance as much as possible.

We might also want to reduce the amount of impact exercises we do, because any moves where we land with force, like jumping, can add extra pressure onto our joints.

How much you need to tailor your exercise will depend on the degree of pelvic girdle pain you experience, but what's most important to remember is that you can still exercise and you should feel confident in that!

Part of the challenge when women are diagnosed with pelvic girdle pain is that some might feel worried about moving altogether. But if we stop moving completely and become immobile, our joints can become stiff, which will only make us more uncomfortable, exacerbating the issue.

We must keep moving. In fact, a new theory of managing pelvic girdle pain actually suggests challenging your mind and body with new movement patterns, which can encourage your brain to respond differently.

Here's how it works. If you've been living with PGP for a long period of time, your brain might begin to anticipate pain with movement, so you may hold back from exercise and become over-cautious, changing how you walk or sit. This could end up making your movements stiff or create imbalance throughout your body if you are overusing other muscles to protect the joints you don't want to use.

It can help if we give the brain a new focus, like walking backwards. In doing so we can help our body practice similar mechanics to everyday activities (like walking forwards), but rewire the brain with the distraction of a new movement pattern. As we're not used to walking backwards, we can focus more on the physical movement than anticipating pain. In this way it's thought that we can help manage the effects of PGP.

PGP reset exercise

● Choose a point on the wall in front of you. You'll need space to walk backwards about 10 steps.

● Keeping your focus on the point in front of you, slowly walk backwards, focusing on foot placement.

● Stop and walk forwards again but as you walk, focus on the point on the wall in front of you.

● Focus completely on that point, walk towards it and tap it twice. Walk backwards again and after completing your steps, walk forwards again, focusing on the same spot. Tap twice and repeat.

● Try this exercise for 3–5 minutes and see how the movement feels. Hopefully your body will have released some anxious tensions and begun to move freely once more.

Women with PGP can also benefit from strengthening the surrounding core muscles to give more support and stability to the pelvis (as in Chapter 4). Exercises targeting the glutes, transverse abdominis and the pelvic floor will be imperative.

If you feel you might be struggling with PGP, speak with your medical team to get their recommendations, and avoid wide-leg stances that over-stretch joints, such as sumo squats and lunges, or single-leg movements that promote pressure down one side of the pelvis.

Ripple effects of prenatal hormones

The hormones we've looked at in this chapter are just a few of the many that fluctuate during pregnancy. The tricky thing is that no one person responds to them in the same way. Some women may notice no significant changes, whilst others find the effects so severe that they experience further repercussions such as water retention or carpal tunnel syndrome.

Water retention

Water retention, also known as edema, might affect you as you move through the trimesters. It particularly affects the legs, hands and feet. Postnatally, it's not uncommon to experience night sweats as our hormone levels settle down and water leaves our system.

My twin pregnancy was the time when I experienced this the most. I guess the double whammy of hormones with two babies heightened my body's experience. But you don't need to be carrying twins to feel it.

For some women, this swelling begins to affect the hands and wrists so much that carpal tunnel syndrome might develop.

Carpal tunnel management

The carpal tunnel is a narrow area of the wrist, through which blood vessels and the median nerve pass. As the blood vessels in the carpal tunnel swell, the median nerve can become compressed, which can cause an ache in the wrist. If you're experiencing this, you might find it helps to introduce stretches for your wrist and forearm. You'll also want to avoid positions that encourage extension of your wrist, like the standard press-up position where your palms are flat on the floor. Some people find that balling their hands into a fist and placing their knuckles down can be a good alternative for some exercises.

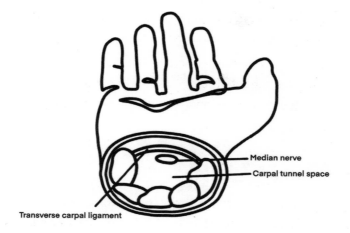

Median nerve
Carpal tunnel space
Transverse carpal ligament

Wrist stretch exercise

● Bring your arms in front of you and place your fingertips together. Lift your elbows out to the side.

● Spread out your fingers as much as you can.

● Now press your fingers towards each other, so that all the fingers touch and your wrists move closer together,

as much as possible. Keep your elbows out to the side. Hold the stretch for a few minutes.

● Move your fingers away from each other again so that just the fingertips are touching.

● Repeat.

Hormones are incredible, aren't they? And now that we have an insight into the changes taking place on a deeper level during pregnancy, in the next chapter we take a quick look at how things change in labour, how we can use the effects to boost our energy during birth, and how our body begins its postnatal recovery.

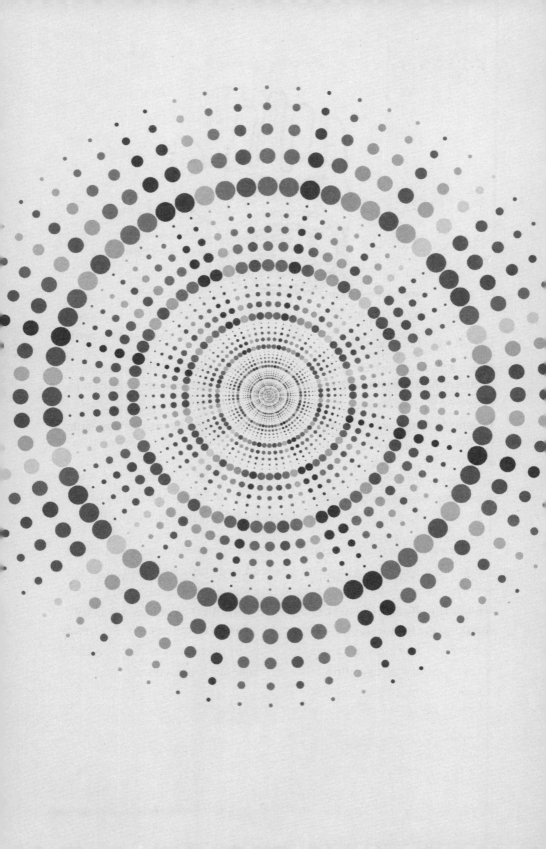

Endocrine system during and after labour

We should all be aware of our endocrine system. Everyone has one, and it's pretty much boss in terms of how our bodies work. It functions in a similar way to our nervous system, except that where the nervous system uses neurotransmitters, our endocrine system has a different messaging system: it uses hormones.

Our endocrine system develops when we're still growing in utero and begins to function even before we're born. It works via a network of glands throughout our body. These glands secrete hormones to regulate many of our body's functions.

We have hundreds of these glands in our body. The hormones they emit travel to different areas, usually via the blood. They then attach to receptors fitting together almost like a key in a lock. Once joined together a message is released, telling the targeted organ what its function is. Things like appetite, blood-pressure control, sleep, body-temperature regulation and reproduction are managed this way.

During pregnancy the ovaries and the placenta are the primary glands responsible for producing pregnancy-related hormones. We've already looked at some key hormones that help our pregnancy to develop and progress, but during childbirth and immediately afterwards we experience more changes still.

Hormones during birth

For labour to progress, two things have to happen. The muscles in the womb need to contract and the cervix needs to soften. Together these two things help your baby descend down the birth canal.

Oxytocin is key to this process. Most antenatal classes will mention this. It's known as the 'love hormone' because its release can be triggered when we activate the sensory nerves in the skin, like feeling touch, warmth and skin-to-skin contact.

It's the feeling we get when we have a new love interest. That spark you feel when you first meet someone and can't wait to be close to them? That's oxytocin!

New couples have actually been found to have high levels of oxytocin. It's said to help deepen and enhance our relationships by encouraging empathy, fidelity and positive communication.

But it's not just about the first flush of love. Oxytocin is crucial in sustaining long-lasting feelings for someone and enhancing positive relationship memories – it has even been linked to the intensity of orgasms.

In labour, when your oxytocin levels rise, it causes regular contractions, which become stronger and more frequent. If labour needs to be induced (brought on artificially), oxytocin or a synthetic equivalent is given to the mother to kick-start the labour process. Oxytocin, along with oestrogen, also plays a part in stimulating dilation of the cervix.

This is why many couples are advised to stay physically connected in early labour, as physical touch encourages things to progress, whether by massage, hugs or stroking. All this can promote oxytocin hormone release.

Postnatally, this hormone triggers the let-down reflex, helping your baby get breastmilk from the breast. This is one of the reasons skin-to-skin contact is encouraged between mum and baby.

It can help to strengthen the bond between you and baby, warm up your body to help comfort your newborn and encourage your uterus to contract back to its original size.

But oxytocin isn't working by itself to trigger these functions.

Prolactin is another hormone we couldn't do without. This hormone is known as a mothering hormone as it's also associated strongly with building the mother-and-baby bond, as well as playing a major role in encouraging breastfeeding.

Levels of prolactin increase throughout pregnancy and peak at birth, falling after delivery. For women who do not breastfeed, prolactin will return to non-pregnant levels within seven days. However, the more we breastfeed or pump, the more prolactin we produce.

Labour is also a time when the role of **relaxin** is crucial. Although levels of this hormone have been produced throughout pregnancy, there's a rapid increase during labour, allowing your cervix and entire pelvic region to soften and expand, making way for baby's arrival!

When labour contractions become more intense, the body also releases a group of painkiller hormones known as 'beta-endorphins'. These are naturally occurring opiates that have a similar effect on our body to synthetic morphine. During pregnancy they play a part in suppressing our immune system, so that it doesn't consider our baby a foreign object and try to fight against it, thereby allowing our pregnancy to progress. During labour, these hormones reduce pain and postpartum they assist with the release of prolactin.

As delivery becomes imminent, the body releases a sudden rush of two other hormones, **adrenaline** and **noradrenaline**. Technically these are known as epinephrine and norepinephrine, but you probably know them as the 'fight or flight' hormones, the hormones that are produced when we're stressed. A rise in these hormones in the later stages of labour will propel us on to continue birthing.

Mother Nature figured that if an animal is close to birth when stress levels rise, such as when a threat emerges, the best option is a swift delivery. When we reach the final stages of labour adrenaline and noradrenaline bring on a rush of energy, making contractions stronger, and helping us to birth our baby quickly.

But if these hormones are released too much in early labour, adrenaline and noradrenaline can work against oxytocin and actually slow things down. In the wild, the release of this pair of hormones can be life-saving. Nature figured that if an animal was suddenly in danger, but it was too early on in labour for a quick birth, the best thing would be for labour to be paused until the mother reached another safe space to continue giving birth.

This is why finding ways to relax and stay positive in early labour is important for expectant mothers.

Many of us will be encouraged to stay at home for as long as possible because this is most likely to help us relax. I, however, felt the opposite. I was much more relaxed when I was in a hospital bed with medical professionals close by. It all comes down to personal preference. If staying at home feels best for you, then run that bath, turn on the tunes and chill yourself into oxytocin bliss!

So how can the knowledge of these hormones help us during delivery?

I imagine you're feeling similar to how I felt when I found all this out. A little overwhelmed and not sure what to do with all the information, but hopefully you're also a little inspired by how cleverly our hormones work together during labour and what a powerful demonstration of love the act of birth is. The way our body, mind and hormones work together to create this near-on magical experience with almost clockwork precision is truly inspiring.

Of course, things don't always go as we expect. As a caesarean mum, I know first-hand how crucial medical intervention can sometimes be in supporting a safe delivery. But the role of our hormones is as important for medicated and assisted birth as it is for natural deliveries. Being able to stay calm amidst unforeseen changes, and overcoming anxiety if we're presented with potential triggers, calls on both our emotional and hormonal systems to kick into gear. Movement and breathing exercises, like the one coming up, can help us to keep calm.

How breathing impacts our endocrine system

Breathing is probably the most common non-drug comfort measure practiced by pregnant women. Many women find it's so powerful that they want to deliver their babies with this technique alone. But even if you opt for other support methods, using optimal breathing techniques in the early stages of labour can help things to progress quickly and encourage us to feel calm through the stages.

Breathing techniques, combined with other relaxation methods such as guided imagery, visualisation, hypnosis or progressive muscle relaxation, can be incredibly powerful. I remember being taught to visualise a balloon floating away with each contraction. With each inhale – then referred to as my 'up breath' – I was told to picture a balloon being filled up with air and, as I exhaled – on the 'down breath' – I was told to picture that balloon being pushed away. But we don't always have the time, or desire, to visualise a scene, and breathing can work well on its own too.

Hypnobirthing expert Siobhan Miller kindly shared one of her favourite simple breathing exercises with me.

Birth breathing exercise

'This breathing technique is an absolute game changer and, best of all, it's so easy to do, it's completely free and you don't need to remember to pack anything – you always have your breath with you!

'Use this simple breathing technique (in for four, out for eight, four times over) every time you experience a surge. It gives you something to focus on, encourages your muscles to relax and open, and ensures you are bringing much-needed oxygen into your body.'

● To do it, simply breathe in deeply through your nose for a count of approximately four. As you inhale, feel your chest rise and your lungs expand as they fill with air. Then, breathe out slowly and gently through your mouth for a count of approximately eight. As you exhale, feel your shoulders drop and your body soften and relax. Repeat this four times.

● If you struggle to breathe out for a full count of eight, you can always modify this so it works for you. Just make sure your exhale is longer than your inhale.

'This exercise takes less than 60 seconds but has a profound impact,' Siobhan told me. 'It actually changes our physiology. It works by down-regulating our nervous system, slowing our heart rate and reducing the amount of adrenaline that we are producing. It's like a shortcut to instant relaxation!'

I wanted to know more about Siobhan's experience with breathing and the endocrine system. What were these physiological changes she was referring to?

'We know that the mind and body are connected and this is especially true in birth,' Siobhan started. 'For labour to progress we want to feel relaxed and produce oxytocin.

'If you are fearful and panicking, perhaps you feel out of control or unprepared and don't have any tools to help, you will produce adrenaline. This will increase your heart rate and your body will enter fight-or-flight mode. Your blood, carrying all your oxygen, will be directed to your limbs, because in the animal kingdom it allows the mother to fight or run.

'Our body pumps blood from areas which are considered "less important" for immediate survival, like our digestive and reproductive systems. Once the blood (and oxygen) to our uterus is reduced, because we're panicking, labour can become more painful, the muscles work less effectively and thus progress will slow. This then becomes a key reason for intervention. If blood and oxygen going to the uterus is reduced, so too is the blood and oxygen going to our baby, which might lead to signs that our baby could become distressed. It's possible to get caught in a cycle where fear leads to increased muscle tension and pain, which then increases the fear and panic.

'But we can avoid this altogether,' Siobhan said, clearly happy to share how breathing can help. 'We can get out of this cycle by trying to relax, which will again trigger our body to produce more oxytocin. Oxytocin not only makes us feel good but also fuels labour and makes our uterus muscles contract. Whatever helps you to feel calm and relax, like breathing and comfort from those you love, will help you achieve this necessary state of relaxation.'

> **WHATEVER HELPS YOU TO FEEL CALM AND RELAX, LIKE BREATHING AND COMFORT FROM THOSE YOU LOVE, WILL HELP YOU ACHIEVE THIS NECESSARY STATE OF RELAXATION.**

How labour leaves us

There are no words that I can use to describe how the birth of a baby can affect us emotionally. It's different for everyone, but whether the moment is calm or chaotic there's certainly nothing else quite like it.

In terms of our endocrine system, as soon as we give birth it goes into overdrive. It's like Piccadilly Circus at rush hour, with a traffic jam down one street and a speeding motorbike gang racing down the other.

'Fluctuating hormones' feels like a drop in the ocean compared to what's really going on. I feel like this is a throwaway phrase, designed more to stop any further questions than to actually provide answers.

Here's a little insight into what's happening.

Let's take a minute to check back in on some of the labour hormones we've looked at so far: oxytocin, prolactin, oestrogen and progesterone. They've achieved a mammoth task of helping to birth our baby (or babies), but they don't hang up their hats yet; there's still a lot of work for them to do.

Skin and eye contact between us and our baby will promote the continued release of oxytocin and prolactin in our body, which can be found in high levels immediately after birth.

Oxytocin helps our womb to continue contracting, reducing the risk of excessive bleeding and helping our placenta to detach and be delivered. Prolactin, on the other hand, is helping to stimulate breastmilk production and oxytocin encourages that milk delivery to the nipple. Both hormones are busy, working together to support the first moments of motherhood.

Oestrogen and progesterone have other focuses. Signalling to our body that the pregnancy is over, they return to pre-pregnancy levels within just 24 hours. This hasty shift can play a role in affecting our mood too. Everyone responds differently to these hormonal changes. Some women feel elated, whilst others are unnerved or overwhelmed. And it doesn't matter how many children you've had, you may respond differently every single time.

I look back on some of my births now and realise that at times I was so overwhelmed that I wasn't fully aware of the decisions I was making or what was being asked of me. Things happened so quickly that I didn't ask questions; I just went with the recommendations, which weren't always what I would have chosen for myself. Fortunately, I had communicated my labour plan and postnatal desires to my birth partner, who was able to communicate on my behalf at times I felt I couldn't make a clear decision myself.

Emotional care for ourselves and our birth partner during and after delivery is so important. For us mothers, our mind responds as the body does; both need a period of time to adjust to the new circumstances. For some women, birth is not the slow and organic process they were hoping for. Whilst medical interventions are fantastic and save many lives, if our animal instincts are interrupted by other procedures, we may feel scared or worried.

The expectation that the post-birth period is full of pure euphoria and delight only serves to make women uneasy if they don't feel this way themselves. In reality, experiencing feelings of worry or unease is actually surprisingly common.

Often referred to as baby blues, feeling down after delivery can affect up to 85 per cent of women, so a big majority!

It's important that we acknowledge that there can be times when this may develop into a more serious condition, such as postnatal depression or postnatal anxiety. As a mother who has experienced the latter, I know that there isn't a hard line that tells us when things have progressed; however, there are some ways we can tell whether we might need more support.

Midwife and author Marie-Louise (@themodernmidwife) offered some great advice here: 'Conditions such as postnatal depression can present in various ways and the early signs can be really similar to those of baby blues. We might feel low, tearful, lacking in confidence, irritable or not finding pleasure in things that we usually would. When it comes to distinguishing between the two, timescale is important. The most common time for baby blues to kick in is around days three to five when our milk changes from colostrum to the longer-term milk if we have chosen to breastfeed. Postnatal depression, however, is usually diagnosed after these emotions have persisted for two or more weeks.'

Having recently become a mother herself, I wondered whether Marie had any personal experience with baby blues that might have impacted how she now works with women herself. 'If I am honest, I cried all day on day five,' Marie admitted. 'Even with the knowledge I have as a midwife, it didn't stop the tears – they just kept flowing! I have always understood the importance of supporting good mental health for new mothers, but I now have an even deeper understanding of how hard motherhood can be, how many hats you need to wear. As a midwife I can clock off a shift but as a mother you never really switch off.'

Marie agreed that encouraging positive hormone release can be imperative to supporting a happy and positive parenthood, but I wondered how, as a midwife, Marie might suggest we do this, if we're already feeling down because of hormonal changes we can't control.

'Have a postnatal plan!' Marie said. 'So many women have a birth plan but it's important that we also think about the immediate postnatal period. I always tell women to ensure that they have a support network. Whether friends, family or neighbours, have people you can call upon and hand over tasks that make you feel overwhelmed. Also, from the beginning try to schedule at least 5 minutes a day to yourself. When I had my baby I was so strict about this. I made myself take 5 minutes to meditate and to do some deep breathing every day. My partner knew that no matter what happened I needed this time. It's about the little things we do for ourselves daily that make a difference overall, and honouring our needs contributes to good mental health for us and our baby. I can't recommend it enough. Self-love and self-care matter in the postnatal period.'

The phrase 'it takes a village' came to mind after I spoke with Marie, and the thought stuck with me for the remainder of the day. Sometimes it might seem as though the process of pregnancy, labour and birth is only happening to us as the mother, but there are so many parts of the journey we can and should share with those closest to us.

As someone who has had a history of anxiety, I remember feeling as though the idea of relinquishing control or being vulnerable would increase my nerves. But coming out the other side, I now know first-hand how the relationships with those closest to us can be instrumental in sustaining our recovery.

Labour and birth are beautiful and challenging and empowering all at the same time. We have seen how much is going on within us, so whilst our body does its thing to begin the recovery process, let us support it further, by taking off some of the pressure when we can and physically and emotionally sharing the journey with others.

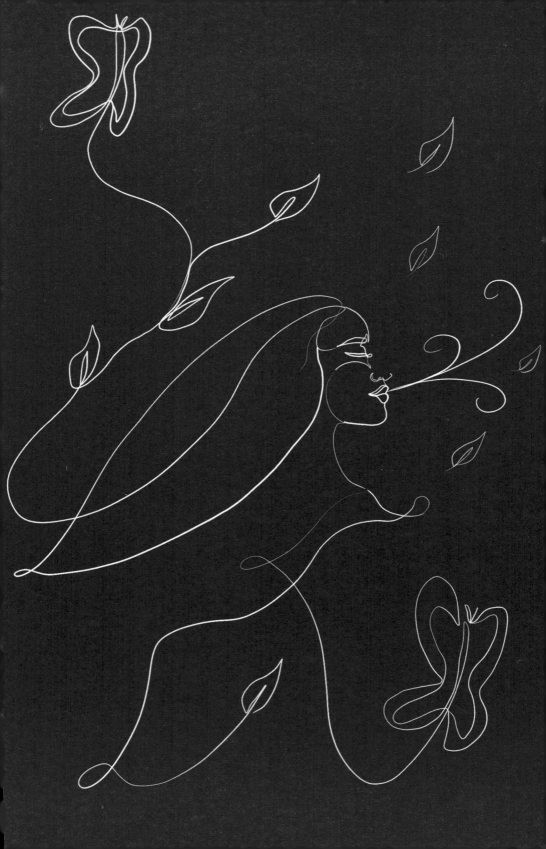

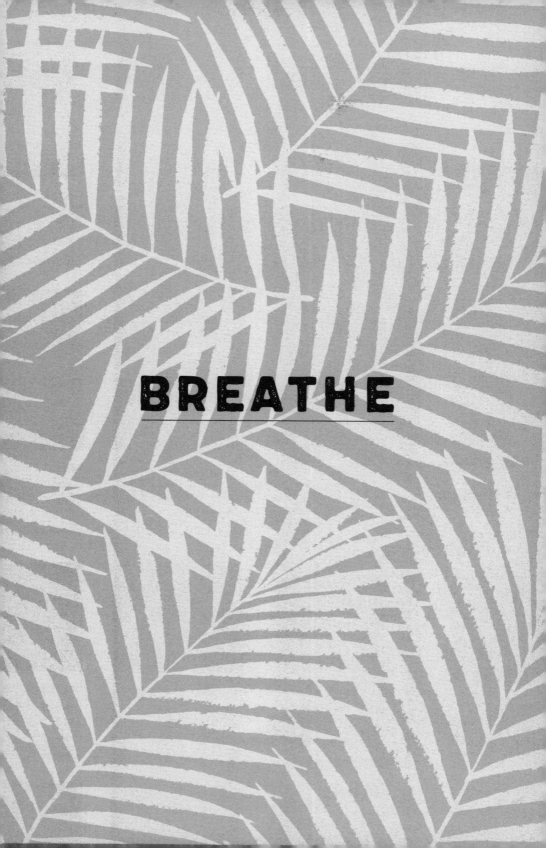

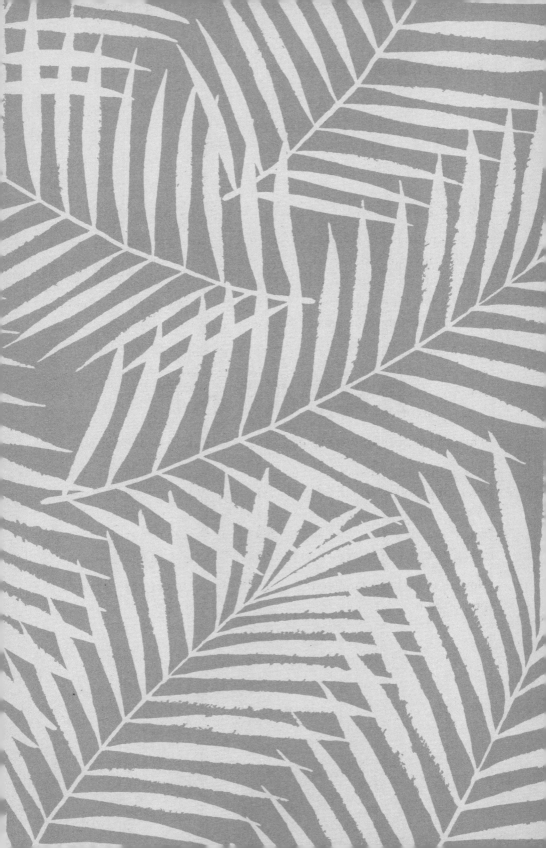

The mind–body connection

Occasionally, memories of those first few antenatal classes I attended pop into my mind. Mostly because now, as a mum of four, I realise how much more could have been said. It wasn't that the information wasn't there. A lot of it was, but without the full understanding, I wasn't taking it in. I like to know *why* I'm doing something rather than just *how*.

For example, I remember being told to practise breathing and relaxation in preparation for labour. The expert leading the session started guiding the group through a visualisation and asked us all to sit still with our hands relaxed at our sides.

This simple instruction filed me with dread. I did not like sitting still.

With a history of anxiety, for me the idea of having to be still was never a relaxing thought. Habitually I was always moving, tapping my fingers or wiggling my toes, so for me the idea of being still and 'just' breathing wasn't calming at all. But I also couldn't deny the benefits everyone else was experiencing from this advice. So I had to give it a go.

Now, as I look back, I understand why this was so important for labour preparation.

Throughout pregnancy, birth and postpartum, the mind–body connection has been proven to be powerful. Research has shown that during pregnancy, negative stress can trigger a hormonal change that passes via our bloodstream and placenta to our baby. Don't panic – a few stressful moments won't cause harm to our little ones, but we do want to reduce prolonged anxiety and stress as much as we can.

Post birth, our mood can filter through to our babies as well. Young children are so in tune with our emotions and energy. Picking up how we feel from our body language, tone of voice and even eye contact, our babies will begin to mirror our emotional state.

I'll admit, my first pregnancy was a steep learning curve when it came to relaxation. I was by no means the ideal mindful role model, and although I'm still not one of those women who can breeze through the trimesters with seeming ease, by the time I gave birth to my twins, six years later, staying calm and relaxed by working on my breath was my main coping mechanism, and it worked wonders!

What changed in the six years between my first and last pregnancies was my understanding of the true depth of the mind–body connection and the power of a good breath!

❛WHAT CHANGED IN THE SIX YEARS BETWEEN MY FIRST AND LAST PREGNANCIES WAS MY UNDERSTANDING OF THE TRUE DEPTH OF THE MIND–BODY CONNECTION AND THE POWER OF A GOOD BREATH!❜

How our body talks

Our skin is our body's biggest sensory organ. It's constantly communicating and inspiring other functions. It talks to our muscular system, our endocrine system and even our emotions. From blushing when we feel embarrassed, or getting goosebumps when we brush someone's hand, to sweating after exercise – these are all ways that our skin communicates with the rest of our body.

The same is true in reverse. If you think of a time when you felt scared, for example, you will notice your heart beating faster or palms beginning to sweat. We don't actually need to be experiencing something to make us scared. Our thoughts and memories can trigger our body into the same response.

Similarly if we feel physically relaxed, we'll notice our minds unwind as well. This is why many relaxation techniques will have you picturing a beach, open field or other happy place.

Just knowing this, however, isn't enough; someone telling us to relax when we feel uncomfortable won't make us feel more at ease. Being able to relax when we encounter stress is something we need to learn and it's hugely beneficial if we can, particularly as we prepare for childbirth. Our body needs to be able to relax under pressure and our mind is the key to doing so.

The stress connectors

When we're stressed our body secretes a certain set of hormones to help us cope, including adrenaline and cortisol. As we know, the main function of these hormones is to make energy more available, so that we can run from a threat or challenge an opponent. The release of these hormones is part of the 'fight or flight' system. Adrenaline, for example, increases our heart rate, whilst cortisol raises levels of glucose (sugars) in our bloodstream. This all plays a part in boosting our energy levels.

Most animals have this trigger and it can be life-saving. The hormones released in this process are also thought to boost our brain function and heighten senses like sight or hearing.

The problem is that in modern-day life we don't just encounter short-term stressors. Unlike other animals, that use this sudden spike of energy to flee from a threat, many humans today encounter stress on a more long-term basis, perhaps due to weeks of broken sleep, difficulties with breastfeeding or trying to juggle a stressful job. If we don't try to find moments to unwind and rest our body enters a state of long-term stress.

Some of the fight-or-flight hormones become depleted, leaving us fatigued and in pain. Alongside this, if we're in a stressed state, we can go without much food or rest. Mother Nature figured that when animals enter a stressed state it's best to stay on the move and not need to rely too much on food or rest. As a result, for modern-day humans, prolonged stress can bring with it negative effects on our sleep, diet and digestion.

Our body begins to feel this stress on deeper levels. Even our pelvic floor health can suffer. For pregnant or postnatal women, this can be hugely detrimental to recovery.

A stressed pelvic floor

That's right, your pelvic floor can get stressed out if you do!

Ever heard people talk about an overactive or hypertonic pelvic floor? That's the technical term for a pelvic floor that won't relax, which is exactly what happens when you're over-stressed.

An immediate trigger of the fight-or-flight response is contraction of our pelvic floor. This is nature's way of preventing any leakage if we need to move fast or escape danger. But when we're put under prolonged stress, continued tension of our pelvic floor can begin to affect our pelvic floor function.

If your pelvic floor is in a constant state of partial contraction, you might struggle to relax these muscles, leading to pain during intercourse, difficulty urinating or incontinence. The pelvic floor can become so tight that it struggles to function at all, and could trigger pelvic organ prolapse.

There are other body areas that become tense with chronic stress too, like clenching our jaw, curling our toes or balling our hands into fists. We know that our pelvic floor is connected along the deep front line to other areas of our body, so tightness in these areas could mean we trigger tension in the pelvic floor as well.

Signs of a stressed pelvic floor can vary from woman to woman, but you might find you have a slow flow or discomfort when urinating, unexplained back ache, abdominal pain, constipation or difficulty inserting tampons.

We've looked at two exercises already that use breathing to relax the pelvic floor (page 39 and page 59), and here's another that also places our pelvic floor into a gentle stretch. Note: prenatal women who aren't comfortable on their back should avoid this position and choose an alternative exercise.

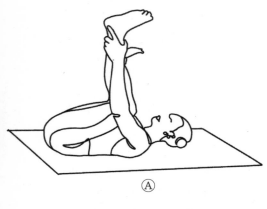

(A)

Breathe in happy baby pose exercise

For women who are prenatal and no longer feel comfortable lying on their back, you may opt to use a bolster or pillows so you're at an angle, instead of straight on your back for this pose. Or you could practise this breathing technique sitting in a chair.

● Lie on your back with your knees bent upwards towards your chest (image A) or supported on a wall if you prefer (image B). If using the wall, hold this position for the remainder of the exercise.

● If you are doing this exercise without the wall, allow your knees to move wider than your chest and then bring them up towards your armpits. You may wish to hold onto your feet or ankles with your hands, but try to keep your ankles higher than your knees.

● You should be creating a 90-degree angle at your knees.

● As you inhale, imagine the pelvic floor relaxing and your diaphragm descending. As you exhale, sigh out the breath through an open mouth. Don't try to tighten the pelvic floor on the exhales. Inhale again and focus on the release of your pelvic floor.

● If you're struggling to let go, visualisation can be a great help. As you inhale, you want to imagine your vaginal muscles opening as well as your rear passage as if you are passing urine or a bowel motion. You can also imagine a rose bud opening until you feel your floor soften.

● You can either hold this position or gently rock on your back from side to side.

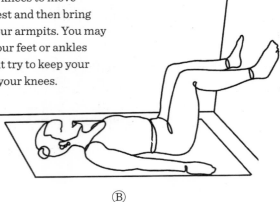

(B)

The vagus nerve response

When we enter fight-or-flight mode, our body has a system in place to help us re-establish calm. This mostly occurs via a long nerve called our vagus nerve. The vagus nerve runs from the back of our neck down our spine and branches out to our heart, lungs, stomach, kidneys, intestines, digestive tract and, in women, our reproductive organs.

The vagus nerve is the main component of a network in our body called the parasympathetic nervous system, which runs communications between our brain and our body. It has some pretty big jobs to do, overseeing our mood, heart rate, immune response, digestive function and generally letting our brain know how our organs are feeling. This link between brain and body makes the vagus nerve a key part of the mind–body connection.

The jury's out on how much the vagus nerve can be stimulated safely (if at all) during pregnancy or labour. Research is still ongoing, but we do know that vagus nerve tendrils send instructions to release hormones like oxytocin, prolactin and another called vasopressin, which can help to calm us down.[12]

Our gut also uses this pathway in the opposite direction, to send messages to our brain via electric impulses called 'action potentials', signalling either stress (fight or flight) or calmness.

The fact that this pathway is a two-way street confirms that our physical body can affect our mindset. Sometimes we just need to let go physically before we can let go mentally, or, better yet, we should practise both together for optimum results!

When I was in the thick of suffering with perinatal anxiety, I was constantly tense. Emotionally I craved control and physically I didn't want to 'let go' at all. My hands were often balled into fists or fidgeting and my jaw was tense. The idea of not being in control scared me. This is also why I found pregnancy and parenting such a trigger for my anxiety.

Not knowing exactly what was going on inside me every single moment was a challenge and something I'm sure some other women will be able to relate to.

But I learned with time that letting go can actually be even more empowering and relaxing than holding on. And sometimes this starts with physical release. If we can release tension in our body, our mindset can follow.

A simple way of relaxing our entire body is the body-scanning technique we looked at in Chapter 3 (page 31), where we travel up the body, focusing on releasing tension. I learned this from Chloe Brotheridge, hypnotherapist and author of *The Anxiety Solution*, when she helped me recover from postpartum anxiety years ago. It's best to do this when you have no time pressure. I preferred to practise at the end of the day when the children were already in bed.

We can also adapt this exercise, by first tensing and then releasing one muscle group at a time. This allows us to be more aware of individual muscles, and focus on the feeling of relaxation in specific areas.

Muscle release exercise

● Lie on the floor or sit on a comfortable chair or sofa if you prefer.

● Relax your body as much as possible and breathe deeply in and out for a few minutes.

● Starting with your feet, tense and then relax individual muscles. For example, curl your toes and clench both of your feet. On your next exhale, completely relax your feet. Continue relaxing them for the next few breaths.

● From your feet, move on to practise the same technique with your calves, hamstrings, glutes, abdominals, shoulders, arms, hands, neck and jaw, each time tightening and then relaxing the muscle group.

● It may feel strange to begin with, but after working each muscle group you will notice an overall sensation of relaxation and calm.

Vice versa

We know this isn't a one-way street. In the same way that physical tension can affect our mindset, our mental state can also have a profound impact on our body.

It might not be often that we consider our thinking cues. Physical pain like a stubbed toe or a stiff neck instantly demands our attention, but for some reason negative thinking, although it can be just as damaging to our health, slips under the radar for months and sometimes years, before we realise just how much of an effect it has on us.

We know from the previous chapter that postnatal depression can present in many forms and is often left undiagnosed for quite some time. Affecting up to 15 per cent of new mothers, this is unfortunately a fairly common condition in the postnatal period.[13] Sometimes being aware of the physical and hormonal changes that our body is going through can have a positive effect on our mood; however, there are times when additional support is needed. If you feel you may be living with postnatal depression or anxiety, please do reach out to your GP or midwife for extra support.

However, even for mothers who wouldn't consider themselves to be living with postnatal depression, negative thinking or self-critical thoughts can be unsettling and unfortunately easily ingrained into our daily habits.

At first it might seem difficult to identify. Have you ever paused to consider what messages you are sending yourself?

Critical thinking cues may include:

- Comparing yourself to others.
- Comparing yourself to your past self.
- Blaming yourself for uncontrollable changes.
- Obsessing over one area of improvement.
- Setting goals that make you anxious or upset, rather than excited.

We can all think like this at times. In fact, often we're harshest on ourselves, judging our own behaviours and actions much more than we would other people's.

It also doesn't help that, as women, we are bombarded by messaging from a very young age telling us that we need to make improvements. This fuels our negative self-talk. I remember being thirteen and feeling out of place because I hadn't waxed my eyebrows yet. These types of expectations, no matter how small, can follow us throughout our lives, and if we let them they can trigger negative thinking patterns.

Becoming a mother can sometimes be a catalyst for even more of this kind of pressure. I remember a friend telling me, 'It was like being catapulted onto centre stage. Never has anyone been more interested in what my breasts were doing, how I was moving or what I was eating or wearing.'

According to data, up to 90 per cent of new mums feel a pressure to be perfect, based on images they see of 'perfect' mums online.[14]

I think we can all agree that trying to achieve other people's stereotyped ideas of motherhood is an unachievable and exhausting task.

Over the years, these attitudes have led women to doubt their ability as mothers and even their ability to birth. But we should never underestimate the power of our body or our own animal instinct.

Hopefully this chapter has shown just how important it is that we prioritise mental wellbeing alongside our physical recovery. Not only is this integral to our overall health, but the benefits of positive mental wellbeing also filter through to our children.

'Happy mum equals happy baby' is a popular phrase and there is truth behind these words. Our babies feed on our energy. Studies have found that babies will show physiological changes of their own that correspond with their mother's stress levels, such as an increased heart rate.[15] This research found that the more stressed out a mother is, the greater the stress response in her baby, a correlation which could become stronger over time.

We know from the start of this book, in conversation with Anna Mathur, that we don't need to worry about a bit of stress or negative emotion. Processing negative feelings is an important part of learning to cope. No one can be expected to feel great all of the time. Blowing off steam and feeling upset are part of human nature and it's in overcoming these moments that we learn that we can cope.

However, taking our mental health seriously means respecting the connection between our body and mind. Our body is always talking to us and our emotional stress may begin to show with physical tensions that inhibit our recovery. We should all feel encouraged to seek extra support if we need it. It might feel confusing or scary at times, but as someone who is now on the other side, I know how important it is to accept guidance and continue to be aware of our long-term thinking patterns.

ACCORDING TO DATA, UP TO 90 PER CENT OF NEW MUMS FEEL A PRESSURE TO BE PERFECT, BASED ON IMAGES THEY SEE OF "PERFECT" MUMS ONLINE.

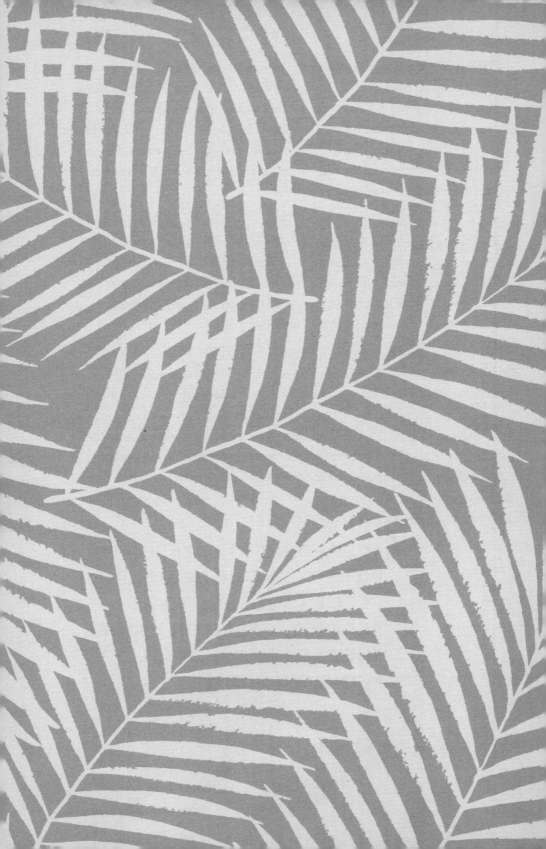

The immediate postnatal period

If you're reading this as a recently postnatal mother, then congratulations are in order. Let's take a minute to contemplate how awesome that is.

If you're still pregnant and waiting for labour day, then let's be clear: you're equally amazing, plus you get my full respect for reading ahead and getting some good preparation done! The last few weeks you might be feeling full of anticipation (as well as quite literally full with baby) but the time will come sooner than you can say 'nappy change'!

This chapter is about the immediate postnatal period, which I count as weeks 0–8 after delivery. It begins as soon as you've given birth. At this point your body changes its focus from creation to recovery. Those first 8 weeks are also when a baby is considered a newborn. Everything is 'new', no matter whether you're a first-time mum or a seasoned professional.

What does your body need in order to recover quickly?

No matter whether you sailed through pregnancy or felt like the 9 months were a struggle, the first 8 weeks postpartum are considered a transition period. That's not to say that come week 8, you'll be fully functional and ready to hit the road running. Full recovery will take many months. Even if you feel you've made huge progress within weeks, there will be deep changes taking place that you can't rush. For many women the healing process may continue for much of the first year, and for some it can take even longer.

Many professionals steer clear of giving exercise advice in the immediate postnatal period, but I think it's important. These early days are possibly some of the most important, when we can ingrain healthy habits. It won't be burpees, but there are a lot of exercises we can do that will benefit us, provided, of course, that we feel ready.

The most important thing for the early postnatal period is that you use your mind–body connection and stay in tune with how your body is feeling. You might not feel ready to exercise yet. Even after the 6–8 week check with your GP, where you may be given the all-clear to progress to exercise, you might not feel ready.

I remember after the birth of my twins, I was given the all-clear to run just 4 weeks after my caesarean section. Against my better judgement I laced up and gave it a go. But it became clear very quickly that my body wasn't up to the task. I jogged for about 3 minutes and stopped to walk home. We need to listen to our body and trust how we feel.

If you're looking for definitive answers about how much exercise is best and when to do it, let me start by sharing some of the latest recommendations. Of course, there's no one-size-fits-all approach to postnatal recovery; you are the best person to know what's right for you, but here are a few guidelines for reference.

General timelines

For many, the majority of postpartum symptoms can ease within the first few weeks, but for others, recovery can take longer.

For those who had a vaginal birth, soreness in the perineal area (the section between the vagina and anus) can take roughly 2–6 weeks to settle down. There is an extended period of recovery for those who experienced an assisted delivery or episiotomy (an incision of the perineum during birth).

If you have given birth via a caesarean section, you'll most likely spend between a few days to a week in hospital following the birth, with further check-ups lasting for up to 6 weeks. Standing, walking and lifting might all feel strange at first, but with the correct rehabilitation exercises, effective rest, sleep and relaxation our bodies will heal relatively quickly.

Regardless of how you gave birth, many women will be cleared for exercise at 6–8 weeks by a GP.

❝THESE EARLY DAYS ARE POSSIBLY SOME OF THE MOST IMPORTANT, WHEN WE CAN INGRAIN HEALTHY HABITS.❞

Perineum recovery

Your perineum is the area between your vagina and anus. This thin layer of skin and muscle fibres lies just in front of your pelvic floor sling. In the third trimester exercises on page 94 we saw a sketch of this region and talked through perineal massage techniques, to help prepare this area for birth by massaging and stretching the perineal fibres.

The speed of perineal recovery after birth depends a lot on the degree of trauma suffered by the area during birth. Healing can take anywhere from 3 to 8 weeks, which I know sounds like a broad scale, but it really does depend on your individual healing process. It may even take a little longer for some women who have had an episiotomy.

Similar to when we massage this area in pregnancy, it's a good idea to get a mirror and take a look at your perineum postpartum, if you feel comfortable doing so. This might make you feel squeamish at first, but often, even though it might feel like a big change has taken place, by looking we can see that only minimal trauma has happened to the area. Understanding the extent of a tear can help us to heal better and make a seamless (excuse the pun) recovery!

Third- and fourth-degree tears

If you've experienced extensive perineal trauma, I would advise visiting a women's health physiotherapist who can assess your personal case. The depth of a recovery can't be outlined without personal one-to-one examination, but thankfully Clare Bourne (@clarebournephysio) has kindly agreed to share her expert advice on how to reduce pain and recover quickly.

1 Warm wash

'After a tear of any degree, taking a glass of tepid water with you to the toilet and pouring alongside your stream, can help to dilute the urine and reduce any stinging sensations,' Clare told me. I actually found this worked so well after my first delivery that I used it as relief during my second birth. At the point of crowning, I asked my midwife to pour some lukewarm water over the perineal area, which helped the muscles to relax and gave the sensation of reducing any stinging when baby's head was crowning.

2 Padsicle

In contrast to the warm-water wash, but equally effective, was Clare's second tip. 'We can create something called a "padsicle",' Clare suggested. 'This is a homemade cold compress which helps to reduce inflammation and soothe the area.'

How to make a padsicle:

- Take a clean sanitary towel and wet it with water.
- Wrap it up in the storage bag it came in or use a freezer bag, thin sterile wrap or face towel to cover it and place it in the freezer.
- Once frozen, wrap in a clean face towel. You can place this over the perineum or stitches for 5–10 minutes at a time. It works just like an ice pack and will help to reduce discomfort.
- Use once and discard. Make a new one and use every few hours if needed.

3 Towel elevation

You might be recommended a perineal cushion, also known as a 'doughnut', by your midwife, which will elevate you when you're sitting down, to help keep pressure off your perineum. 'I'd often recommend something much simpler,' Clare said. 'A doughnut can work for some people, but for others the shape of a circle can actually put their perineum into a stretched position as they sit on it. Instead I'd suggest simply rolling up two towels and placing them parallel to each other, so that as you sit down they are placed along the length of your thigh. Sitting in this way means that you will still relieve pressure on the perineum by being raised off the seat, but without there being any "tugging".'

4 Refuel to repair

One of the first things we can access to help us recover is what we eat. Anything we put into our system effects how our body behaves. Even our hormones are impacted by our diet.

'You want to really look after your bowels,' Clare explained, 'because hard or backed-up stool can increase pressure on your perineum or caesarean incision.'

Thankfully, gut health is becoming a much more prevalent topic of conversation. In fact, the power of the gut is so important that it's even now referred to as our second brain. We know from the last chapter that our gut communicates with our brain via the vagus nerve, and providing our bodies with a variety of healthy vitamins and minerals can have positive effects on our brain function, mood and stress levels.

We'll be covering nutrition and gut health more in Chapters 13 and 14 but Clare did have a useful tip for the immediate postnatal period. 'Try to include lots of fibre in your diet,' Clare recommended, 'as this will help your stools to be a good consistency which helps to make them easier to pass.'

Not only will an efficient function of your bowel help alleviate pressure on your perineum, it will also help to prepare your body for your first postpartum poop.

Being anxious after surgery to pass a bowel motion is actually very common. I'm sure most mothers will agree that the idea of bearing down on an already vulnerable area is less than inviting. I barely suffered any tearing in my first delivery but for some reason was still nervous about going to the loo. We can literally scare ourselves shitless, and as ridiculous as that might sound, this hesitation means that constipation can be common for new mums.

'But holding on will only exacerbate the issue,' Clare told me. 'The longer stool stays in the bowel, the bigger and harder it becomes, which can lead to constipation, putting extra pressure on the pelvic floor, which is something we want to avoid.'

Many women are offered a laxative after a third- or fourth-degree tear, to help them pass their first motion with ease. 'You can also create a basic splint to support this area when you need it, such as when passing a motion,' Clare suggested. 'Use a clean sanitary towel, maternity pad or simply wrap toilet roll around your fingers and hold this against your perineum as you pass a motion.'

Often women can be asked to limit their fluid intake before birth, particularly if medication is required, so after delivery we want to make sure we rehydrate again, which will also help our stool to move.

Turns out, there is actually an optimum poo position as well, that is incredibly effective!

OPTIMUM MOTION POSITION

● Sitting on the toilet, place your feet up onto a stool, so that your knees are resting higher than your hips.

● 'Lean forwards in this position to help the pelvic floor relax and the bowel to become straighter, opening up the back passage, creating a sort of slide, and *weeeee*–!' Clare said with glee. 'The poop can ride out!'

5 Self-care

'Self-care of the perineum is, of course, so important as well,' said Clare, as professionally as if we hadn't just been discussing a poo slide. 'Along with any medication you might be taking for pain relief, there are many healthy home habits we can do to help our recovery too. The vagina is very good at keeping itself clean, but we want to make sure we're changing pads regularly and freeing up the area completely as often as possible. By allowing fresh air to reach the wound we can encourage the healing process to happen naturally.

'A good daily routine,' Clare recommended, 'is to have a shower, with gentle water pressure, avoiding soaps. Simply let the water wash over the area. Then take a towel and lie on the bed or floor, with legs open and free, to allow air to get to the area.'

6 Exercise and perineal recovery

'Movement is good, little and often as it can help us manage swelling,' Clare advised. 'Any one position, sitting or standing, for too long, can become uncomfortable. Movement helps us alleviate that.'

Gentle pelvic floor exercises might be far from your mind in the early days, particularly if you've had a perineal tear, but as soon as you feel ready, these can be started postpartum, even within a few hours provided your catheter has been removed and you have successfully passed urine.

'Re-engaging the pelvic floor will allow you to regain some control over the muscles and feel them working again,' Clare said. 'It may be that things feel a little different, but becoming reacquainted with the area is important to recovery.'

Pelvic floor activation

In order to activate our pelvic floor muscles properly, we want to aim for global activation, which means engaging all pelvic floor muscles together.

Historically, pelvic floor exercises were taught as short sharp squeezes, as though you are 'stopping the flow of urine'. But it's now widely agreed that to activate our entire pelvic floor, we need to visualise a much bigger movement. This exercise begins with a deep inhale, as with the three-dimensional exercise on page 39, but this time we will activate our pelvic floor muscles more by using a new visualisation that allows more complete engagement of the pelvic floor on the out breath.

The visualisation part of this exercise involves picturing our coccyx bone at the back of our pelvis coming together with our pubic bone at the front. We should visualise these bony structures moving inwards, towards one another, and then drawing upwards together along the midline.

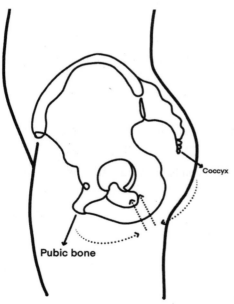

Coccyx

Pubic bone

● Lie back on the floor with your knees bent and feet flat on the floor. This exercise can also be done seated if this is more comfortable for you. Keep your legs hip-width apart. You may choose to support your head with a soft block or pillow.

● Breathe in and visualise the three dimensions:

1 Expansion of the rib cage.
2 Allowing the air to fill your torso by the sensation of pushing your back into the floor.
3 Relaxation of your pelvic floor.

● As you exhale, draw up the pelvic floor by visualising your coccyx bone (at the back) and pubic bone (at the front) coming together and lifting up. Count to eight and focus on the visualisation throughout.

● Inhale and relax your pelvic floor, working through the three dimensions again.

● Repeat the visualisation on the exhale.

- Remember to keep your shoulders relaxed throughout. If you notice them lifting, it is a sign that you're not inhaling fully, so relax and start again.

- You may wish to place your hands low down on your belly, just above your pubic bone, to feel the pelvic floor activating. To find the right position, take your forefinger and middle finger on both hands. Place them on the hip bones either side of your waist, then walk the fingers 2cm inwards and 2cm down. This should be around the pubic bone area. Focus on feeling the deep core muscles engage on the exhale.

Lochia

Lochia is the technical term for postnatal bleeding, which can last for up to 6 weeks. It is made up of leftover blood and tissue from the uterus and will be heaviest for the first week to ten days before slowly decreasing and tapering off around the 6–8 week mark. We want to make sure Lochia has stopped before engaging in certain exercises like swimming.

Diastasis recti

As mentioned in Chapter 4, diastasis recti happens in 100 per cent of pregnancies by the time baby is due. It refers to the separation of the two halves of your rectus abdominis muscle, and is crucial to allow room for your bump to grow.

Although every single mother will experience diastasis recti to some degree, there still seems to be a lot of stigma around this condition and many worry about how they'll recover.

The truth is that for some women the gap will come back together on its own by the 6–8 week check with their GP. However, more than half of us will be diagnosed with this condition after our 6–8 week GP check.

The general guideline is that a gap wider than 2cm is something you should raise with your medical team, who might want to run further investigations. A gap smaller than 2cm can be rehabilitated with exercise.

We can actually assess the size of our gap ourselves. If you have any concerns, it's always best to run them past your medical team, but here's how to self-diagnose how big your own gap is.

Diastasis recti self-assessment

● Lie on your back on a flat surface.

● Place the soles of your feet on the floor so that your knees are bent. Keep your feet hip-width apart.

● Place one hand under your head for support and place the index finger and middle finger of your other hand onto your sternum. This is the top of your midline (image A).

● Curl your head off the floor but keep your shoulders relaxed.

● Holding this position begin to walk your fingers down the midline towards your belly button.

● Feel for the sides of your two rectus abdominis halves.

● If you find a gap, try rotating your fingers so that they are lying side-by-side in the crease of the gap. Each finger is roughly 1cm wide (image B).

● If both fingers fit into the gap and there is still room to spare you should speak with your GP about further assessment.

● If both fingers fit in the crease side-by-side without any additional room, continue with core rehabilitation exercises, such as those in Chapter 10.

One of the first signs of diastasis recti can be a bulging or a dipping in at the midline. If you're performing an exercise which involves contraction of your abdominals, like a plank or sit-up, and you notice a raised path pushing out from your midline, it could indicate that your deeper core muscles, like the TVA and pelvic floor, are not creating enough tension to support your core in action. This can often happen around the belly button but also occurs above or below. The exercises coming up in Chapter 10 can help to build the strength of our deep core muscles.

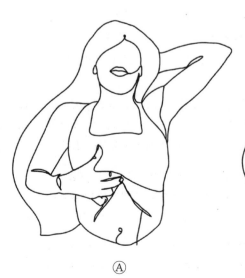

Ⓐ

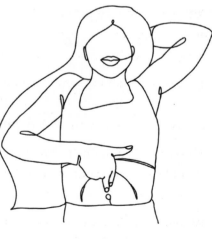

Ⓑ

Caesarean recovery

Many women I have met have voiced concerns about feeling overwhelmed by the recovery after a caesarean section. There seems to be a lot of confusion around how we should be healing and what we can expect when returning to exercise.

As a caesarean mum myself, I know first-hand that it can be frustrating if you feel as though recovery is moving too slowly. Simple movements might feel strained to begin with. I remember telling my husband after that first week that I felt alien in my own skin. Tasks I previously hadn't struggled with now felt difficult, which I found upsetting, and I had to work hard to stay motivated.

Alongside the physical changes, we also have a visual wound to get used to which can create triggers of its own on a deeper level.

There are simple measures we can take to help scar tissue recovery on a deeper level and reduce the outwards signs of our scar as well. How we move, feel and even what we eat all play a part in how this scar tissue behaves.

❝BREATHING, MEDITATION, WALKING AND MINDFULNESS HAVE ALL BEEN PROVEN TO REDUCE STRESS AND ARE SAFE TO PRACTISE IN THE EARLY POSTNATAL PERIOD.❞

The incision from a caesarean heals from the outside in, meaning it can look healed on the outside when there is still a lot of recovery to be done underneath. Skin is a fast healer, knitting together a new framework within just a few days or a week. But the further in we move through our body's layers, the longer the wound takes to come completely together.

Scar tissue itself is formed slightly differently to our natural skin. Although it might feel tough or rubbery to touch, it actually only ever reaches 70 per cent of the strength of the muscle it's replaced. Internally, scar tissue can also continue to develop, twisting around other organs or binding soft tissue structures to other internal tissue.

It's even thought that emotional stress can trigger scar tissue regrowth, which highlights how important it is for us to remain positive and relaxed throughout recovery. Breathing, meditation, walking and mindfulness have all been proven to reduce stress and are safe to practise in the early postnatal period.

Breathing and scar tissue recovery

I never believed that breathing alone could have a direct impact on my postnatal recovery, but it absolutely can! If you're rolling your eyes, let me share with you how.

I mentioned before that by taking a deep breath, we encourage our diaphragm to descend. The downwards movement of our diaphragm triggers an internal massage of our intestines and other organs, which means our abdominal scar tissue is kept mobile.

Scar tissue massage

This is something we can start at 6–8 weeks postpartum. By this time the wound covering should have been removed (hopefully with a little more compassion than mine was!) and the wound has healed. I was shocked to find a swollen 'pouch', around my scar after the covering was taken away and it didn't seem to be reducing much over the first few months. Again, I turned to Clare for some advice and we started working through the massage techniques below. I soon noticed big improvements.

'We should be working on a completely healed scar,' said Clare. 'There should be no scabs. If you've had an infection of any kind, that can delay your start time, so don't just take the 6-week guideline as read. Also, if at any time you don't want to work directly onto the scar, you can still begin by massaging the skin around it.'

Before starting any of the following exercises, we should first make sure that we feel emotionally ready to be hands-on with our scar. Having a strong emotional reaction to your scar may take you by surprise, and feeling uneasy about manipulating the skin around the incision is very common. Clare shared with me some insights from her professional experience: 'Initially, some women may struggle to touch their scars. If massage brings on any emotional feelings, flashbacks or post-birth trauma I'd always advise that you stop the massage and seek further support.'

When you are ready to begin, start with a few minutes a day and progress up to 10–15 minutes at a time, a few days a week. Our skin is a highly sensory organ, so the simple act of stimulating the skin allows for a calming and cortisol-lowering effect which helps healing. The hands-on mobilising of the area also increases blood flow which helps to speed up recovery.

1 CLOCKWISE CIRCLES

Begin on the middle of your abdomen, placing two or four fingers just below your belly button. Use gentle circular motions, all the way down to just above the scar, in a clockwise direction to encourage blood flow and mobility of the area.

2 SIDE TO SIDE

Using two or three fingers, positioned directly above the scar, where you can begin to feel some tension, work a slow side-to-side motion, almost as though you are rubbing the scar, but slowly and with control. Once you feel ready this movement can be performed on the scar itself, still using two fingers side to side.

3 SCAR MOBILITY

Once you feel confident you can begin to rub small circular motions on the scar in a clockwise motion.

Following on from this, use two fingers next to each other to move the scar up and down, taking the slack on the skin and gently moving it over and back across the scar.

4 SCAR STRETCHING

It may take a few months for you to feel confident manipulating the scar in this way, but once you are ready you can place two fingers either side of the scar to gently stretch the scar tissue and surrounding skin.

Begin by placing your index fingers and middle finger close together but either side of the scar. Slowly move the fingers away from the scar in the centre, one up and the other down, so that the scar and surrounding skin is stretched.

5 PICK UP AND PINCH

At a similar time to the above exercise, you can begin to 'pick up' the scar and roll it between your fingers.

For this exercise use your thumb and forefinger. Place them either side of the scar and gently pinch the skin together, lifting the scar away from your skin.

In this raised position, rub and roll your fingers together and roll the scar tissue in the process. Slowly lower and move along the scar to repeat in a different location.

Underrated rest

Rest is seriously underrated, even by some medical professionals. But getting enough rest and sleep is imperative.

Rewind fifty years and it wasn't uncommon for women to stay in hospital for up to 2 weeks or longer after delivery. Your baby would have been brought to you for feeding and whisked away again so that you got enough rest.

Whilst I can't say that I'm hankering for those olden days in other respects, the idea of prioritising rest for the mother sounds wonderful.

I had to give sleep its own chapter – it's simply too important to squeeze into a few paragraphs – but here's a snippet of the basics.

When we sleep, our general energy consumption is lowered. Imagine your body as a steam train and your energy as the train driver, shovelling coal into the fuel tank. When the train is on the move, the driver (our energy) is focused on pouring coal into the tank. The faster the train moves, the more fuel we need. It's only when the train stops and the engine is no longer needed, that the driver (our energy) can focus on re-energising and refuelling herself.

When we sleep and our brain and body are mostly at rest, we can put more energy into repair and regrowth. This happens via an increase in the production of growth hormones and blood flow.

It's via our blood that oxygen and nutrients are transported around the body. When we are being active our blood delivers more oxygen to the working muscles to give them energy. But when we sleep our body can turn more of its focus on repair and regrowth as opposed to using the energy to move and think.

I know, I know… even the idea of getting quality sleep when you have a newborn is something of a pipe dream. In fact, I write this on the back of a night's 'sleep' where the twins woke up every hour from 1am onwards!

But let's not panic just yet. Whilst sleep is the best way, it isn't the only way for your body to recover. Research has shown that rest can provide us with similar benefits to actual sleep. It's not exactly the same, but sitting down and relaxing still allows our body to adapt to the stress of a busy day. In short, sometimes make sure you prioritise having a sit down; your body needs it!

❝REST IS SERIOUSLY UNDERRATED, EVEN BY SOME MEDICAL PROFESSIONALS. BUT GETTING ENOUGH REST AND SLEEP IS IMPERATIVE.❞

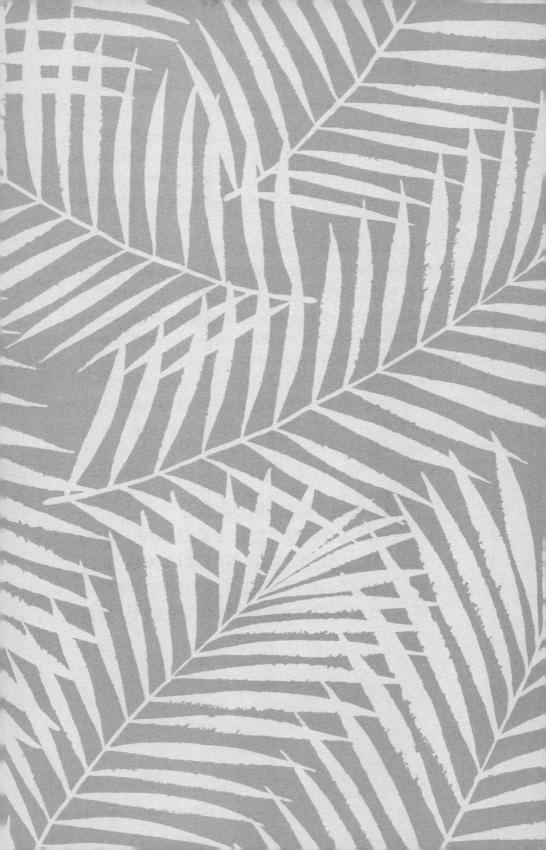

Exercises for weeks 0–6 postpartum

Ah, weeks 0–6. The period of time where I like to claim that giving birth exempts me from needing to wash dishes, unload the dishwasher or answer emails on time. Not because I can't, but because I've been such a hero at delivering life that I can now pick and choose which household chores befit my new station of superhero!

Ideally, I'd meet every one of you super-mamas too. Not only to congratulate you, but so we could have a one-to-one review of your pre-pregnancy and pregnancy health, as well as details of your labour, birth and postnatal experience, because ideally, all of this is needed before giving you specific exercise advice.

But whilst a face-to-face chat isn't possible, I'm hoping that all the information in this book will give you a good insight into what's right for your body and understanding how you feel. Because exercise in the first few weeks postpartum is entirely down to just that: how you feel.

I mentioned already that the current guidelines say that where pregnancy and delivery have been uncomplicated, exercises like pelvic floor work and walking may begin immediately after delivery. However, this by no means guarantees that every woman will want to engage in exercise during this time.

Generally it's safe to assume that at some stage during the first 6 weeks, you will be up on your feet and, when you are, even if you're just moving around a little, it's important that you have healthy movement patterns in place to help support and strengthen your body for what's next.

Here are my top ten exercise suggestions for the immediate postnatal period.

Some of these moves might seem super simple, but these exercises will give us the building blocks to lay strong foundations for future workouts.

> **IT'S IMPORTANT THAT YOU HAVE HEALTHY MOVEMENT PATTERNS TO SUPPORT AND STRENGTHEN YOUR BODY FOR WHAT'S NEXT.**

1

Reconnect with your breath

The below is a great way to reconnect with your breath postpartum and encourage synergy between your respiratory system and deep core. This is also the base for rehabilitating diastasis recti.

To prepare

● This exercise can be done seated, standing or lying flat.

Place your hands onto your lower abdomen if you can, just below your belly button so that your thumbs are in line below your belly button and your index fingers create a V shape pointing diagonally downwards towards your pubic bone. You should now be creating a triangle shape in the middle of your hands.

● All three points of the triangle should be level with one another; this indicates that your pelvis is in a neutral position.

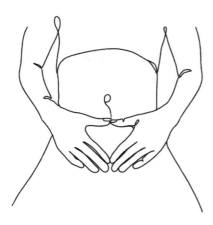

To perform the exercise

● Take a deep inhale and feel your belly expand into your hands, keeping your shoulders relaxed. Allow your ribcage to expand and pelvic floor to relax. This isn't bearing down but just a relaxing of your pelvic floor muscles.

● As you exhale, gently breathe out through your mouth as though you are slowly blowing out a candle. Simultaneously draw up the pelvic floor by visualising the pubic bone and coccyx coming together and lifting up, as in the pelvic floor exercise on page 149.

● Focus on keeping your pelvis in a neutral position throughout this exercise, bracing the pelvis. The three points of the triangle should be level.

● Exhale slowly for a count of eight.

● Inhale and release your pelvic floor, allowing your diaphragm to descend and ribcage to expand, keeping your shoulders down.

● Repeat this deep breathing technique for a few minutes, inhaling for a slow count of eight and exhaling for a slow count of eight also, if possible.

2

Lying pelvic tilt

This exercise is great to reconnect with your pelvic floor and deep core muscles. It's one of the first exercises we can use to recover diastasis recti and rehabilitate a weakened pelvic floor, whilst continuing to encourage optimal breathing technique.

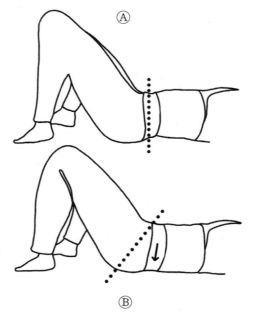

● Lie back on a flat surface, with your knees bent and the soles of your feet flat on the floor (image A).

● Keep your feet hip-width apart, with your arms relaxed by your sides.

● Inhale and relax your pelvic floor, filling up your belly with air and keeping your shoulders relaxed and down.

● As you exhale, draw up your pelvic floor by visualising your coccyx and pubic bone coming together and lifting up.

● As you engage your deep core muscles, allow your pelvis to gently tilt backwards, connecting your lower back to the floor (image B).

● Hold this pelvic tilt for the duration of your exhale, eight counts if possible.

● Inhale and release your pelvis back into a neutral position, relaxing your pelvic floor simultaneously.

3

Pelvic tilt progression with march

This exercise is a good progression on the lying pelvic tilt.

● Lie back on a flat surface, with your knees bent and the soles of your feet flat on the floor. Keep your feet hip-width apart, with your arms relaxed by your sides.

● Inhale and relax your pelvic floor, filling up your belly with air and keeping your shoulders relaxed and down.

● As you exhale, draw up your pelvic floor, simultaneously tilting your pelvis backwards, as in the previous exercise, connecting your lower back to the floor.

● As you tilt your pelvis, lift one foot off the floor, bringing your knee towards your chest.

● Aim to exhale for a count of eight.

● Inhale and lower your foot back to the floor as you release your pelvic floor and return your pelvis to neutral alignment.

● Repeat the exercise, lifting the other leg.

● Continue alternating legs for 10 repetitions each side. All marches should be performed slowly and with control.

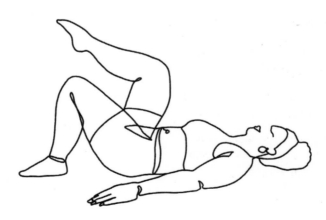

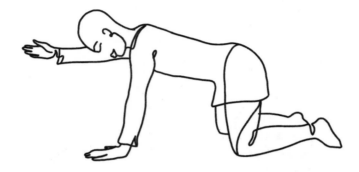

4

Four-point arm raise

This exercise will target the pelvic floor and deep core muscles, encouraging them to work in synergy.

● Begin in the table-top position with your wrists, elbows and shoulders stacked in a straight line, shoulder-width apart and your knees under your hips, hip-width apart.

● Inhale and relax your pelvic floor.

● As you exhale, draw up your pelvic floor and raise your right arm off the ground straight out in front of you. As you do this, focus on maintaining good alignment along your spine, keeping your hips level, without tilting.

● Inhale and return your right hand to the floor.

● Repeat on the other side.

● Continue alternating hands for 8 reps each side.

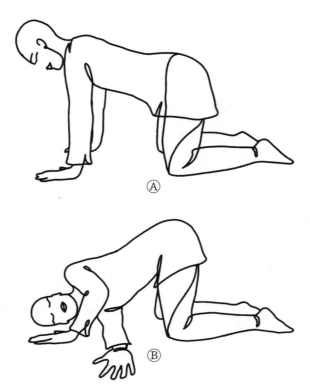

5

Thread the needle

Stretching is often underrated and under-practised but postnatally it becomes even more important. This exercise helps open up the shoulders and mobilise the spine which is important to support a fully functioning core.

● Start on all fours, in the table-top position, with your wrists, elbows and shoulders stacked in a straight line, shoulder-width apart and your knees under your hips, hip-width apart (image A).

● Inhale and lift your right hand off the floor a few centimetres.

● Tracking your hand with your gaze, follow your hand as it moves down and through, underneath your left arm.

● Sink into the stretch by keeping your hips high but allowing your chest to lower down towards the floor. Keep some pressure in your left palm to avoid crunching your neck and allow your right shoulder to brush the floor if possible (image B).

● Hold this position for a few deep breaths then push through your left palm and raise your chest back up to the start position, placing your right palm back on the ground.

● Inhale and repeat on the other side.

6

Standing foot relaxation exercise

Stretching and releasing tension in our feet will also encourage release of tension in the pelvic floor.

● Face the wall and stand a foot back.

● Place the toes of one foot against the wall.

● Lean forwards a little until you feel the arch of your foot stretch. Take a few deep breaths and allow yourself to gently relax into the stretch.

● Repeat on the other side.

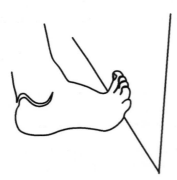

7

Jaw relaxation exercises

Similar to our feet, relaxing our jaw will encourage the release of tension in our pelvic floor.

● Sit or lie in a quiet, relaxed place.

● Take a deep inhale and place your tongue on the roof of your mouth.

● As you exhale release your jaw, allowing your mouth to open slightly.

● Breathe in and out for a few breaths, allowing this relaxation to deepen.

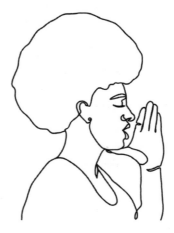

Progression

● When you're ready, take one thumb and place it under your chin.

● Open your mouth so that you feel some resistance against your thumb.

● Hold for 3–6 seconds, then close your mouth slowly and feel the release.

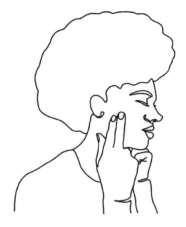

Jaw massage

● To massage our jaw and encourage further relaxation, take two or three fingers from each hand and place them onto the masseter muscles, either side of your jaw. They are found directly behind your molars, just below your cheekbone. It's one of the main muscles used to open and close the jaw when chewing.

● Gently press your fingers inwards and move in a circular motion for a few minutes.

8

Chest doorway tension release exercise

It's common for chest muscles to become tight, particularly for breastfeeding women, who often adopt a posture of rounded shoulders when nursing. This stretch allows us to open up the chest and encourage good alignment.

● Stand in the middle of a doorway.

● Bend both of your elbows to a 90-degree angle and lift your forearms so that they rest on either side of the doorframe.

● There should also be a 90-degree angle at your shoulders but be aware not to hunch your shoulders up to your neck and instead keep them relaxed and down.

● Take a step forwards with one leg, through the doorway, so that you feel a stretch on your chest muscles.

● Focus on pulling your shoulder blades back and down.

● Hold for a few deep breaths and step back to a neutral position.

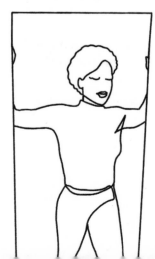

9

Kneeling hip flexor stretch

Our hip flexor muscles are a group of muscles that attach at either our lumbar (lower) spine or pelvis, extending all the way down to our thigh. They can become strained during pregnancy as our pelvis shifts and our belly grows, creating an arch in our lower back. This posture can have several consequences and might leave us with back pain or feeling as though we need to stretch our hip flexors postpartum.

● Kneel on a mat, using a chair, bench or sideboard for support on one side if needed.

● Bring your left foot forwards, bending your knee to a 90-degree angle so that the sole of your left foot is on the floor. You should now be in a kneeling position on one side with your right knee down (image A).

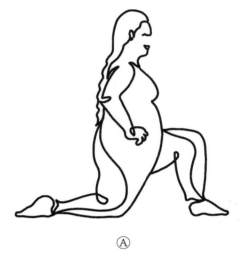

(A)

● Inhale and as you exhale, slightly tuck your pelvis under to lengthen your lower back as you simultaneously shift your weight forwards through the front leg. You should feel a lengthening in the front of your hip on the left side (image B).

● Hold for a few deep inhales before slowly bringing your right knee back onto the floor, returning to the start position.

● Avoid overarching your lower back throughout.

● Repeat on the other side.

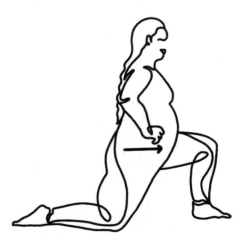

(B)

10

Sitting-standing combo

Functional training refers to exercises that help to prepare us for everyday movements like sitting, standing, reaching, lifting and walking.

● Sit on the edge of a seat with your knees bent and your feet aligned just behind your knees, the soles of your feet flat to the floor. Keep your legs hip-width apart. Relax your arms by your sides (image A).

● Inhale and as you exhale, gather up your pelvic floor and push through the heels of your feet as you come to standing.

● Once standing at full height with your knees straight but not locked, take a deep inhale.

● On the exhale, bend your knees to sit back down on your seat, whilst drawing up the pelvic floor once again.

● Once you are sitting down, inhale and relax your pelvic floor.

● Exhale and repeat the movement. To progress this exercise, as you push through your heels and come to standing, simultaneously reach your arms up and extend them overhead (image B). Return your arms to your sides as you bend to sit back down.

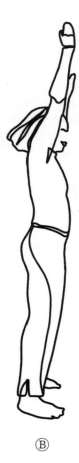

Ⓐ

Ⓑ

Postnatal posture checks

Once in a while, it's a good idea to check in with how we are naturally sitting and standing, and giving ourselves a few prompts to engage the correct muscles and achieve optimal alignment.

Here's a quick debrief on how our posture should be when we're sitting and standing.

Seated posture check

● Sit on a chair, with your back straight and your shoulders relaxed and down.

All three natural curves of the spine should be present while sitting. This includes the cervical curve by your neck, the thoracic curve by your torso at chest level and the lumbar curve at your lower back. You may wish to use a lumbar support or roll up a small towel to support your lower back. Just be aware not to create so much pressure that your back is placed into an overarched position.

● Make sure that your body weight is even across your hips, distributed between both sitz bones.

● Your knees should be bent, in line with or just higher than your hips.

● Keep the soles of your feet flat to the floor.

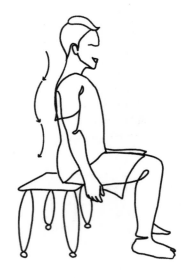

Standing posture check

● Stand up tall with your feet placed shoulder-width apart.

● Bear your weight primarily on the balls of your feet (not on your tiptoes).

● Keep your knees straight but not locked.

● Your arms should relax naturally down at your sides.

● Allow the natural three curves of your spine and keep your shoulders relaxed down and backwards.

● Keep your head level. Your earlobes should be in line with your shoulders. Avoid pushing your head forwards or backwards.

Holding any static position for too long, whether sitting or standing, can begin to compromise our posture and lead to aches and strains, so try to stand up often and take breaks if you're sitting for long periods of time. I've lost count of the hours I spent nursing in those early postnatal days, but standing up and working on a few mobility shoulder rolls, chest stretches and deep breaths was a great way to reset and recharge.

If you are standing for long periods of time you might want to rock back and forth on your feet or move slightly from one foot to the other to alleviate any building tension.

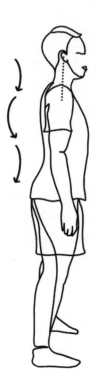

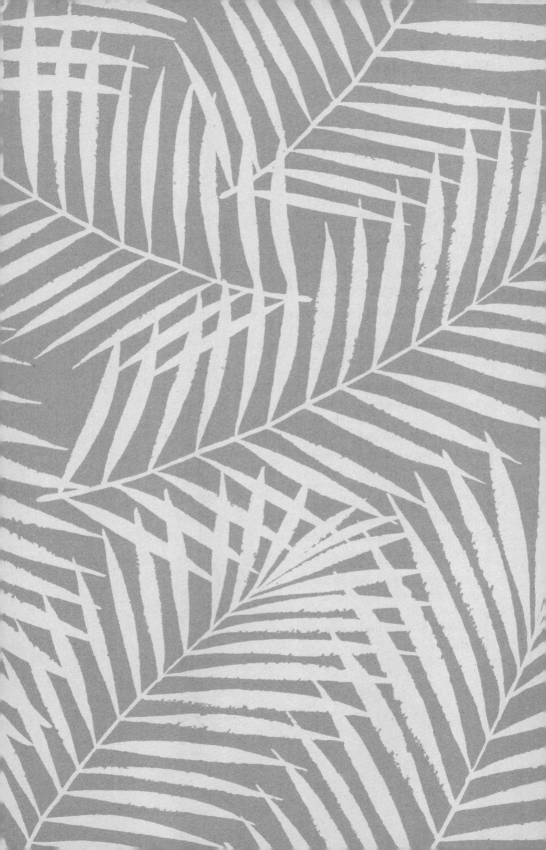

Rest, recovery and quality sleep

We've been through a few key elements of recovery now and got started on our immediate postnatal exercises. But alongside keeping active, getting enough rest is also imperative to recovery.

It's said that laughter is the best medicine but if something was to contest that it would be sleep, because it's pretty much a wonder drug. No super-green, organic, gluten-free, natural, kefir, avocado, health substance can beat it!

When we sleep our body focuses more on healing and strengthening. Some of the greatest benefits from a workout happen after the exercise has taken place. When we're at rest, this is when our body can consolidate all the elements of learning and strengthening it has done throughout the day, and recover stronger and more efficiently. This is actually why we sleep more when we're feeling unwell. Our body needs the extra rest in order to focus on making us better as quickly as possible.

Without taking rest days and getting adequate sleep, our body won't function at its best and neither will our mind. Our brain needs sleep just like our body. It's during sleep that our mind can transfer information from short-term memory to long-term, and refine tasks like motor and sensory development.

Babies sleep a lot (except when we need them to, right?). This is because their brain and body are developing at an incredible rate. A baby is born with only approximately 25 per cent of its adult brain, but by three years old this has increased to 80 per cent. That's a lot of learning!

As for adulthood, I don't know about you, but I LOVE to sleep. Don't all adults?

During pregnancy and post-birth, craving sleep can become even more prevalent. When our body has more of an energy demand placed on it, like when we're growing a baby, we need more rest. Increased stress or mental pressures, like a new job or any complications that could arise during pregnancy, also cause our body to crave more rest.

I don't want to sound like I'm questioning Mother Nature here, but, in my opinion, evolution missed a trick with sleep and parenting. How is it that no matter how much sleep we might want, our nights during that first year of motherhood are almost always interrupted?

If we need sleep to assist with the release of the growth hormone, encourage muscular repair and boost brain function, why can't we new mums seem to get enough of it? How are our bodies meant to recover efficiently if we're constantly having broken nights' sleep?

Well, ladies, let me introduce you to sleep's BFFs, 'rest' and 'napping'. For those of us that can't manage a full night's sleep, let's get better acquainted with these two.

The power of sleep

Not to rub your face in what you're missing, but let me quickly outline the power of sleep.

Our sleep cycle works in four stages.

Stage one lasts only a few minutes and consists of the initial moments from when we close our eyes to when we drift to sleep.

Stage two lasts around 30 minutes, during which our body temperature lowers, our muscles relax and our heart rate and breathing become more regular. During this time, sleep spindles become active. Spindles are waves of activity, assisting lots of actions like memory consolidation and cortical (brain) development of motor, sensory and visual functions.

Then we enter stage three, where we move into what is known as slow-wave sleep. This lasts about 20–30 minutes and is when we're in our deepest sleep. This is where our brain begins to convert and transfer information from short-term memory to the long-term. It's during this stage that we might struggle to wake up most (and, sod's law, probably when our babies decide they'd like a night feed!).

The fourth stage of sleep is when our brain becomes more active again. It's known as rapid eye movement sleep (REM). We might find it easier to wake up from this stage of sleep than the third. REM sleep is a time where our inhibitions and cognitive control are lowered whilst other areas of the brain, like those associated with emotions and motivation, become more active. It's thought that this is where bizarre dreams come from. With our inhibitions lowered, our brain is free to create wild associations.

Exactly how long each stage of sleep lasts can vary depending on the time of day, and from person to person too. It's even possible for our cycles to change from night to night based on a wide range of factors such as our age, recent sleep patterns and alcohol consumption.

Generally speaking, if a sleep cycle is roughly 90 minutes (1.5 hours) long, and our baby is waking up every 3 hours throughout the night, like many newborns do, that means that between 10pm and 7am every other sleep cycle we're woken up. On average it's believed that during the first year, parents will lose about 109 minutes of sleep every night.

But don't despair! Napping can help to keep us on a healthy track.

Nap hacks

It appears that there's pretty much a 50–50 split between those of us who nap and those who don't. Many debates have been had on the best length of time for a nap, to ensure we reap the benefits, but science is showing us that there can actually be multiple answers.

The most suitable one for motherhood, I think, is however long you can get!

Ever heard of the 20-minute nap theory? We've tried this in our house, mainly because it seemed like an achievable amount of time when the babies might also stay asleep. The idea behind this is that we never enter that third stage of deep sleep. Napping for 10–20 minutes allows us some benefits from stage two, but as our body hasn't entered deep sleep yet we should, in theory, be able to wake up without too much trouble. I tried it a few times though and wasn't totally convinced. I found that I would still sometimes wake up exhausted.

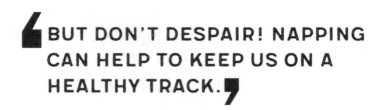

BUT DON'T DESPAIR! NAPPING CAN HELP TO KEEP US ON A HEALTHY TRACK.

It turns out that time of day plays a big part too. Humans are meant to sleep at night; we're not set up to be nocturnal. We don't have night-time vision or a heightened sense of smell or hearing. When it's dark, our body knows it's time to sleep. This is set by our 'circadian rhythm'.

You might have heard this phrase thrown around in relation to sleep. We all have a circadian rhythm, and it's led by the light and the dark.

Interestingly we aren't born with circadian rhythms, which is why newborn babies have such erratic sleep patterns. There's no light in the womb, so babies need to develop their circadian rhythms after birth, usually by around 6 months of age. Which is when, hopefully, they begin to sleep for longer periods.

We actually have a few circadian rhythms working internally on 24-hour cycles, which all help to form part of our 'body clock'. Along with setting our sleep-wake cycle, this also helps our body regulate appetite, body temperature, hormone levels, alertness and blood pressure.

It's our circadian rhythm that makes our body feel 'off' when we travel to a different time zone. It needs time to adjust. While we're falling asleep at the holiday bar at 4pm, our circadian rhythm is hard at work resetting night and day.

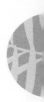

There are other biological clocks working in our body as well but for different lengths of time. The infradian rhythm, for example, works on a longer time frame and is responsible for our menstrual cycle.

When it comes to sleep and napping, our circadian rhythm plays a big part, but it's only half the story. There's something else working alongside this that helps regulate our sleeping habits. It's called 'sleep drive' and it's basically our body's natural urge to sleep.

Our sleep drive works opposite to our circadian rhythm. Whilst our circadian clock is using the light to help us stay alert, our sleep drive is building up throughout the day, pushing us towards sleep. The longer we're awake the more our sleep drive gains power and begins to pressure us to sleep.

When we sleep we regain our natural energy balance. The fancy name for this is homeostasis. And once our body has achieved homeostasis, the pressure from our sleep drive diminishes. The morning comes and the light tells our circadian rhythm we're ready to wake up. This explains why our energy can be low on grey, cloudy days. Our circadian rhythm feels out of sync due to the lack of natural sunlight.

So how does our circadian rhythm relate to our naps?

As mothers, sometimes all we can do is grab what rest we can when the opportunity hits, but if we can, research suggests that morning or early afternoon are the best times to nap and feel refreshed for it.

Napping in the late afternoon is where trouble sets in. This is because napping partially diminishes our sleep drive so sleeping too late in the day could affect our need to sleep when night comes.

Here are some quick tips on how to ensure you have the best nap!

Set an alarm

This is essential. We don't want to oversleep with a nap. The best length of time is either 10 to 20 minutes, or up to 90 minutes so we enter stage four REM sleep, which is easier to wake up from than stage three. Just remember that longer naps may affect your overall night-time sleep.

Nap early

Napping too late can interfere with our nightly sleep. Try napping in the morning, even if you feel energetic, to prepare yourself for a busy day ahead. At the latest, schedule your nap for halfway between when you wake up and fall asleep in the early afternoon.

Set a sleep environment

Try to avoid using technology in the time before you nap, and take a few deep breaths to help relax your body and mind. Find a quiet and comfortable place to help yourself fall asleep and feel relaxed when resting.

De-stress

Try to release any mental worries as well. Mental stress can hinder our ability to fall asleep. If you struggle to let go of your thoughts, try some relaxation exercises like square breathing.

Square breathing exercise

- Sit in a chair or find a comfortable space to lie down.
- Take a few deep breaths and relax your body a little more each time.
- Close your eyes and when you're ready, begin to use your breathing to assist you in drawing a square with your mind.
- Inhale and visualise one side of the square, drawn straight up in front of you.
- On the next exhale visualise the top line of the square moving horizontally across the top.
- Inhale and visualise drawing the next vertical line down the other side of your square.
- Exhale and complete the square by visualising the bottom line drawn across and touching the bottom of the first line.
- Repeat this visualisation, using slow and controlled breathing throughout. Focus only on drawing the lines of the square.
- Practise this for about 5–10 minutes.

Hopefully these tips will be helpful in giving you a good-quality nap but it would be a little unrealistic to assume that this is always possible. If it's too late to sleep and you find yourself flagging in the afternoon, let's look at how best to reap the rewards of rest.

Relaxation

I know, rest might not be a word we automatically put together with motherhood, but they can co-exist in harmony!

I always find my energy levels dip just before the dinner–bath time saga begins. No matter how well I've slept, around 3–4pm my eyes begin to droop. Turns out I'm not on my own: many people experience this tired period, and it's not exclusive to motherhood. It's so widely experienced that it's even been dubbed the 'afternoon slump'.

It's actually caused by our circadian rhythm and internal body clock. Alongside directing our sleep-wake cycle, our circadian rhythm triggers hormone release that steers our body's natural energy flow, spiking and dipping throughout the day.

The 'main' cortisol peak, which gives us a shot of energy, is estimated between 8–9am, making us feel alert for the day. Smaller cortisol peaks happen again at roughly midday–1pm and 5:30–6:30pm.

The 'slumps' can occur in the gaps, the afternoon slump taking place roughly between 2 and 5pm.

From what we know of our sleep drive, this is far too late to actually sleep without affecting our night-time routine, so here's a quick energy-boosting exercise, and it only takes 3 minutes.

This exercise involves us raising our legs up onto a low platform such as a step or chair. We do this to encourage more return blood flow from our lower extremities (our legs). This means that blood from our legs can be redistributed around our body. Walking around all day means that gravity can cause more of our blood to hang around in the lower half of our body but when we lie in this position, gravity will help our blood to flow to other areas. As our blood is being transported, oxygen is moving around too, giving us more energy.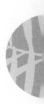

If you are pregnant you can perform this exercise seated. Sit against a wall and raise your legs up in front of you on a pillow or low stool. This smaller angle won't create the same effect as lying flat, but it will still be beneficial.

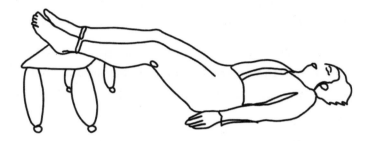

Recharge in three exercise

● Lie with your back flat on the floor, arms by your sides if you can but it's not imperative (half the time I'm holding a baby when I do this). What's important is that we elevate our feet off the floor. This doesn't need to be by a lot; we can use a chair or bench, or even just a pillow if the other options aren't available.

● Take a few deep breaths in this position and be as relaxed as possible for 3 minutes. Deep breaths will encourage more quality O2 in your bloodstream. *Voila* – an instant energy boost!

Everyone should be able to find the time for this 3-minute movement, no matter how busy we are, but if you've got yourself a couple of extra moments, there are some other things we can do to give ourselves an energy boost.

To make our rest even more effective we need to let go of three things: stress, worries and expectations.

Somehow rest has become synonymous with laziness. For a long time I placed a lot of expectation on myself to 'do more'. Any moment that I wasn't parenting or working seemed wasted. But it's actually the opposite. Rest is imperative for life!

It helps our brain to function more efficiently for the day. So we're definitely not wasting time, we're actually investing in improving our brain function, which probably saves us time in the long run.

Letting go of stress and worry can be trickier, but it's not impossible. A counselor I saw in my early twenties once suggested that I try pausing my worrying, which seemed like a funny concept but did actually work when I gave it a try.

'When we're over-stressed or feeling incredibly anxious, it can sometimes help to set a "worry window",' the therapist told me. 'Try to choose a time of day where you allow yourself to worry. Something like, every day at 4pm for an hour, or after your children go to bed. If a worry occurs to you at any other time of day, write it down and wait until later. When that time comes you can focus your mind on your concerns and journal any feelings or angst, but often when it finally arrives, you may feel as though you no longer need it. That's not to suggest that we can never be concerned about something, but feelings of overwhelming anxiety should be left until this time frame.'

I was skeptical but gave it a go and funnily enough I found that my anxiety greatly decreased.

If you do feel as though negative thoughts may be hard to dismiss, we can also use the mindfulness square breathing exercise from page 180, which is useful in helping to shift our focus away from a stressful thought when we need to.

Happy hydration

Being dehydrated will affect our energy. Our bodies need water to survive and even when we're not pregnant, a high percentage of our cells are made up of water. Not consuming enough fluids affects our memory, energy, movement and mood.

Reading signs of dehydration can be trickier than you might initially think. You might even confuse dehydration with signs of hunger. Often, if you're craving sugary foods, your body is in fact signalling that it's low on fluids. Signs of dehydration can include fatigue, lightheadedness, a growling tummy, headaches or dry mouth and lips.

If you're tired, check that it's not due to a lack of water. We should always try to be aware of how much we're drinking every day. There's a good chance that you'll have moments of dehydration and this needs addressing.

Our nutrition can affect our energy levels too. As modern-day humans we've done a good job of confusing our natural eating habits by opting for the 'easy options' to allow for our busy schedules.

But heavily processed foods can zap our energy as our metabolism needs to use more energy to break down and digest the nutrients.

For many, an initial go-to for an afternoon energy boost might be chocolate or caffeine but foods made up of high levels of sugar can also have negative effects on our energy in the long run. We'll tackle more on nutrition in the next few chapters.

Self-care

Rest needs to be a priority and not just 'squeezed in' when we absolutely can't take any more. Reaching burnout comes with its own set of issues, some of which can lead to long-term health complications.

Oftentimes it's assumed that mums put themselves low down on their priority list and research is now backing this up, with one survey showing that 78 per cent of women admit to often putting off taking care of themselves or getting their health appointments made, because they are so busy taking care of other family members' health.[16]

I mentioned before that research is showing that our children will pick up on our stress and their stress response may kick in as a result. Making the above logic that many mums seem to live by ... well, illogical!

Taking care of ourselves not only boosts our own health but also supports that of our children and wider family network.

Similar to exercise, try finding a rest that you enjoy. Read, write, listen, sleep, dream ... However you choose to unwind, rest comes in many forms; what's important is that we have a moment to breathe deeply and relax both physically and mentally.

TAKING CARE OF OURSELVES NOT ONLY BOOSTS OUR OWN HEALTH BUT ALSO SUPPORTS THAT OF OUR CHILDREN AND WIDER FAMILY NETWORK.

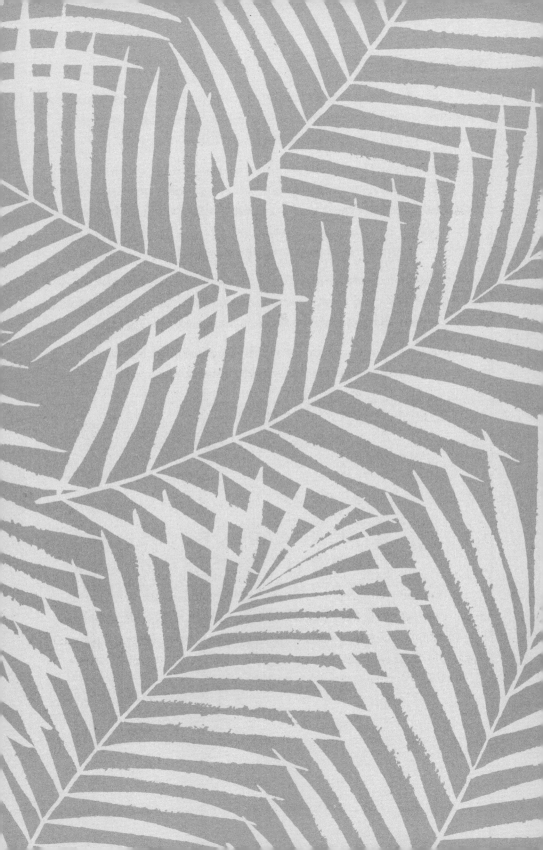

Exercise and breastfeeding

I remember the topic of breastfeeding coming up a lot in discussion with other ladies, even before I had given birth the first time. But, whilst all the technical aspects were covered, the emotional side and the physical effects it can have on the body weren't mentioned at all. Let alone any insight into the struggles we might sometimes encounter.

There was even a poem read out at the first antenatal class I attended, written entirely from the baby's perspective about how much they love breastmilk and how special it is. Although I have chosen to breastfeed my children, it doesn't necessarily mean it will always be the right choice for everyone. There are many benefits of breastmilk, but I can't help feeling that the decision to breastfeed is sometimes forced onto mothers. I'm all for arming women with the facts but there's a fine line between encouraging a mother to persevere, and force.

Overwhelming mothers with information doesn't sit right with me, and if I'm honest, this poem felt more like propaganda than guidance.

Yes, breastmilk is wonderful but rather than reading flowing poetry about how much baby will value breastmilk, maybe we should focus our efforts on sharing the facts and considering how this experience can be for the mother. Perhaps we could even attempt to prepare ladies as much as possible, for any challenges that they may face. Can I suggest a little more reality, a little less Shakespeare?

Breastfeeding and emotional effects

Not all women will choose to breastfeed, and some of those who do may find that they are unable to continue in the way they had hoped. But even women who maintain a long relationship with nursing can at times meet challenges.

When my eldest was born, I thought I knew what to expect from feeding. I anticipated that breastfeeding might not be straightforward, but I wanted to try, and happily I found that my milk came in as expected, no difficulties with latch (unlike some of my other children).

However, I was surprised to find that after the first few days I began to struggle emotionally with the constant demand and amount of feeds my baby needed day and night. I became overwhelmed by the amount of time I spent breastfeeding. No one had prepared me for that.

I felt it much more invasive of my personal space than I had anticipated, and although I loved the closeness with my child, feeding 'on demand' felt almost as though I was being pressured or bullied into it. Add sleepless nights into the mix and I began, quite quickly, to resent the process rather than enjoying it.

Of course, it's not all doom and gloom though. Many women love the experience of breastfeeding and perhaps many more would if they were adequately prepared. I had a much more positive experience nursing my second child, which I did for over a year, and then with the twins, where demand was doubled, I had my most positive nursing journey so far.

I put this all down to being adequately prepared. The second time I knew what to expect and I also knew that those early days, where feeding felt relentless, did pass and a routine of sorts began to take shape.

This chapter is about exercise and its effects on breastfeeding, but be assured that it's perfectly natural for breastfeeding to throw up a range of emotions for you as the mother. Perfecting the latch and maintaining supply are important parts of supporting this process but emotional support is equally important.

I found expressing a great way to give myself a small break, without needing to worry about my baby being hungry, but this again comes with a commitment and being tied to a pump for a period of time. However you choose to feed, know that there are plenty of options for you to explore and discuss with your medical team. Coming up is advice on how to balance breastfeeding with exercise but hopefully along the way you'll pick up a few nuggets to prepare you for nursing a newborn too.

Exercise and its effect on breastmilk supply

I'm asked a lot about how exercise and breastfeeding relate to one another. Can working out have a negative impact on our breastmilk supply, for example?

This subject alone seems to be shrouded in myths, with no one too sure about what exactly is true or false. Actually, the answer is simple, so here goes.

Breastfeeding mamas, please take heart in knowing that exercise has no known harmful effect on yourself, baby or breastmilk supply.[17] YAY!

However, although *supply* is not compromised, the *content* of breastmilk may be altered slightly after higher-intensity exercise. These changes are only temporary though and still considered safe.

For this reason, some women prefer to express before exercising, so that they can use the expressed milk to feed baby immediately after exercise, before levels have reset. Personally I've breastfed straight after exercising and never had cause for complaint. In fact, I've breastfed during exercise on many occasions too – trust me, it's doable!

How is milk content affected?

There are two main changes to breastmilk content after higher-intensity exercise. The first is a decrease in levels of IgA, which is an antibody that plays a role in mucosal immunity for the baby.[18] These levels are decreased ever so slightly but replenish again within 30 minutes. The second is an increase in levels of lactic acid after high-intensity exercise, but this will settle back down to its usual levels after 90 minutes, and, again, there are no known harmful effects to mum or baby.[19]

Some women are concerned that exercise might alter the taste of their breastmilk and make it unpalatable for baby, but there is no research to support this. I would always recommend wiping down the breast after exercise anyway, just to make sure that no sweat is clinging to your nipple which could be an unusual taste for your baby.

What else do we need to know?

While exercise itself might not impact breastmilk supply, dehydration can; breastmilk is almost 90 per cent water! Every baby has varying needs in terms of how much breastmilk they want, so each of us will produce slightly different amounts too, meaning our fluid intake will also fluctuate. Here's a rough guideline for how much milk we will be producing at any given postnatal stage.

- By day 5, a woman may produce around 200–300ml per 24 hours.
- By day 8, 400–500ml per 24 hours.
- By day 14, up to 750ml per 24 hours.

Thereafter anything between 750ml and 1 litre per day can be expected. For mothers of twins, it can be common to produce up to 2 litres, or more.

With so much breastmilk being produced, it's no surprise that we need to increase our fluid intake as well. Our body will give us lots of signals to say it's dehydrated. Feeling thirsty is, of course, one, but there are others too.

Signs you need more fluid can include dry skin and mouth, feeling dizzy or tired, constantly craving snacks or sweets, constipation, dark-coloured urine or suffering from headaches.

To work out how much water you need to be drinking when breastfeeding, a rough estimate would be that you need the amount of water you were consuming before pregnancy plus the increased demand we've just laid out.

Exercising can increase our body's demand for water even more. In order to stay hydrated it's important that we sip fluids regularly throughout the day, which is more effective than a fast intake of a large amount immediately before or after a workout.

Why else might supply be low?

Dehydration isn't the only cause for a decrease in milk supply. Feeling unwell or having high levels of cortisol, brought on by stress, can also affect our breastmilk production.

Once we begin substituting some breastmilk feeds with solids when weaning, our supply may also change to fit the new demand. Researchers believe that breastmilk production works on a supply-and-demand basis, so even when supply feels low, it's recommended that we continue breastfeeding or expressing milk when we can to encourage the demand to build up. If low levels of breastmilk continue, speak with your healthcare team to investigate further and discuss other options. I'm a strong believer in feeding whichever way works best for you and supports your and your baby's wellbeing. If breastfeeding is causing you high levels of anxiety or stress, then you should feel confident in exploring other options and those around you can support you in that decision.

When it comes to feeling under the weather, or catching a virus or bug, this itself won't impact your breastmilk supply; however, related symptoms such as fatigue, decreased appetite, diarrhoea or vomiting can impact milk production. We should continue nursing if we can and supply should settle back to expected levels once we recover. However, depending on how quickly we recover or if any other medication is necessary, we might again need to discuss alternatives with our team of experts such as our midwife or GP.

Diet also plays a part in breastmilk production. I am often asked whether restricting calorie intake can affect breastmilk supply, and the answer is that it can. If we reduce our calorie consumption with the aim of losing weight faster, it can be counterproductive to our milk supply and actually our entire postpartum muscular recovery. It's important that we make sure to refuel with enough calories to support our body as it recovers. We need energy for our body to move, think and heal, as well as meet the demands required for milk production. We don't need to 'eat for two' but an average of 500 extra kcal a day is recommended for breastfeeding mothers.

WE NEED ENERGY FOR OUR BODY TO MOVE, THINK AND HEAL, AS WELL AS MEET THE DEMANDS REQUIRED FOR MILK PRODUCTION.

Does breastfeeding help or hinder weight loss?

I'm asked this question quite a lot, and I can understand why. Some people will swear that breastfeeding is responsible for most of their postnatal weight loss, whilst others profess that they only started to notice a decrease in body fat after they stopped nursing. The actual answer to this question lies in the middle of the two.

In the first few days after delivery, breastfeeding can help to trigger uterine contractions, which themselves play a part in reducing the appearance of our mid-section, where our bump previously expanded. It's also true that breastfeeding burns a large number of calories.

But there are a few things we aren't considering with this first train of thought. Firstly, while breastfeeding burns a lot of calories, it also requires a lot of calories in the first place to maintain a good supply. Along with this, our body also needs to retain some levels of body fat in order to support breastmilk production.

It's not uncommon for breastfeeding women to notice that after an initial drop in weight, which occurs for all women after the birth of baby, placenta and amniotic fluid, they do hold on to a small amount of body fat for the duration of exclusive breastfeeding. Levels may then begin to decrease steadily as baby is weaned from the breast. Interestingly, there are quite a few anecdotal accounts of breastfeeding mothers finding that they particularly notice that they retain increased levels of body fat in their upper body, mainly the arms.

If you want statistics and cold hard facts, research has shown that whilst the rate of weight loss for breastfeeding mothers may be slightly faster than for non-breastfeeding mothers, the results didn't significantly differ.[20] What's most important is that we bear in mind that all fitness goals take time. We shouldn't feel pressure to give up breastfeeding purely to lose weight.

Invest in your chest!

Never underestimate the value of a good sports bra. Our breast size can increase up to two or three times during lactation, which will have a huge effect on how our body moves and feels during exercise.

According to sports physiotherapist Deirdre McGhee, Ph.D, if unsupported, the average range of motion for breast-bouncing can be 3–5cm. Ouch! But a high-support bra can cut this range in half, reducing the uncoordinated bouncing and helping our breasts to move in synergy with our torso. A good sports bra can also help to avoid chafing.

Does breastfeeding affect exercise?

The relationship between breastfeeding and exercise isn't just a one-way street. We hear a lot about how exercise affects breastfeeding, but very little about how it works in reverse. There are some things to consider though, about how breastfeeding can impact our physical ability.

Firstly, as breastfeeding mothers we may find that our posture becomes affected, as we regularly adopt a forwards or rounded position with our upper back and shoulders whilst nursing our baby. An old dance school friend of mine, Grace Hurry (@gracehurrypilates), now a pilates instructor, gave me a great postnatal upper back exercise to help counteract this postural deviation during my early breastfeeding days.

This exercise involves a form of back extension, which can be controversial for postpartum women, as we don't want to exacerbate any abdominal separation by excessively arching the back, which could place pressure on the front of our abdominal wall. However, Grace was clear:

'Upper back extensor activation is different to a full back extension. Upper back activations are a small movement and can be incredibly beneficial for posture support, provided we get the technique correct. It's important that we think more of lengthening our head forwards, rather than lifting our back upwards, which may encourage movement into a middle or lower back arch, and which should be avoided in the early postpartum stage.'

This exercise is best performed after your 6–8 week check, and we should always make sure we have been cleared for exercise by a medical professional. Women with an excessive diastasis recti may wish to postpone this movement until they have fully recovered or achieved a functional diastasis recti. 'To take pressure off your core,' said Grace, 'this movement can also be performed standing, which may be the best option for anyone who considers themselves a beginner.'

❝WE HEAR A LOT ABOUT HOW EXERCISE AFFECTS BREASTFEEDING, BUT VERY LITTLE ABOUT HOW IT WORKS IN REVERSE.❞

Postnatal posture pilates

● Begin by lying on your front, with your arms extended along your sides, fingers pointing backwards, palms facing inwards.

● Rest your forehead on the floor. Inhale to prepare and hover your forehead a few centimetres off the floor.

● As you exhale, draw up your pelvic floor and imagine knocking a marble with your nose gently along the floor a few centimetres. Lift your eyeline up a little and simultaneously stretch your fingertips backwards, drawing your shoulder blades towards your pelvis.

● As a result, your chest will lift slightly off the floor, but this should be a minor shift. Focusing on ensuring that the lower back stays lengthened and relaxed not arched, keep your neck long and reach the crown of your head forwards.

● Inhale and release back to the start position. Rest your forehead on the floor.

● Repeat for 8 reps of slow and controlled movement.

Modification: Upper back activation exercise (standing)

If lying on your stomach feels uncomfortable, this exercise can also be done standing against a wall.

● Stand tall, facing a wall with your chest resting on the wall, arms by your sides.

● Inhale and as you exhale, engage your pelvic floor, drawing your shoulder blades down and towards each other. Simultaneously stretch your fingertips down towards the floor and imagine rolling a marble up the wall with your nose a few centimetres.

● Focus on ensuring that the lower back stays lengthened, not arched; keep your neck long and extend the crown of your head upwards towards the ceiling.

● Inhale and release back to the start position, resting your forehead on the wall.

● Repeat for 8 reps of slow and controlled movement.

Posture isn't the only way that breastfeeding can affect our exercise though. We should also be aware that breastfeeding mothers will continue to produce the hormone relaxin longer than those who don't. If you need a reminder, this hormone is the one that loosens the ligaments in and around our pelvis in preparation for birth but it can affect the rest of our body too. The effects of relaxin will continue to be felt in our body up until about 5 months after we stop breastfeeding.

The increased laxity of our joints means that we need to be careful not to overload or overstretch when we're exercising. We might also notice that the speed and force with which we can move is reduced.

In order to transfer power across our joints, we need stability, so we should take care when doing sudden movements like jumping, sprinting or throwing. We can still enjoy these exercises but we should be aware that our body is coping with higher levels of relaxin and be mindful with our movements.

Interestingly, relaxin is actually released during our menstrual cycle as well. Once our cycle starts again postpartum, we should be aware of its effects at certain times of the month. Relaxin levels begin to increase just after ovulation to prepare our body for pregnancy. If implantation does not occur, relaxin levels drop again until we ovulate in the next cycle. And this isn't the only way that our menstrual cycle can affect our exercise.

The menstrual cycle and its effect on exercise

Ever wondered why you have moments in your menstrual cycle where you feel like you can take on the world, when other days you just want to curl up in a ball under the duvet and sleep? Well, we can all point the finger at our endocrine system – again! Because it's the changes in our hormone levels that cause our energy to fluctuate throughout the month, and this affects how our body responds to different types of exercises during our cycle.

Your period has two phases: the follicular phase, starting from the first day of your period, lasting from day one to day fourteen; and the luteal phase, running from the time after ovulation to the day before your period begins; days fourteen to twenty-eight, roughly, depending on the length of your cycle.

At the start of your period, days one to six, there is a drop in progesterone and oestrogen. This happens as our body sheds the lining of the uterus, and it can be common to notice a dip in our energy at this time.

As we approach ovulation, in the middle of our cycle, there is a surge of oestrogen and testosterone, while progesterone levels stay stable and low. This is when we are at our most fertile, and the surge in oestrogen and testosterone also boost our mood and prompt a rise in our energy levels, allowing us to train more easily.

Many believe that during these first fourteen days a woman's body is able to digest and utilise carbohydrates more efficiently too, which would mean that we have more fuel in the tank to lift, carry and run.

The second stage of our cycle, the luteal phase, are the days between ovulation and the start of our period. During this time oestrogen and serotonin levels decrease and it's progesterone levels that start to rise.

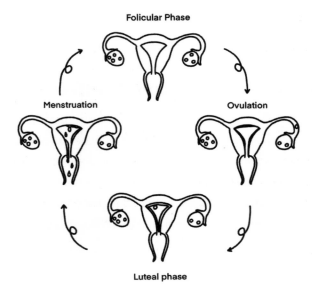

As we near the start of our period we might begin to feel our energy take a knock. Generally, progesterone is seen as a mood depressant, as opposed to oestrogen and serotonin, which give us a natural lift. So, as these levels rise, we might find we're more tired and fatigue more easily with exercise.

That's not to say that we need to skip training or that we can't set and achieve goals at all times of the month. Athletes have been winning events and achieving personal bests throughout all stages of their cycle, but taking into account the hormonal changes in our body is useful to understand how and why we feel a certain way.

As for when our menstrual cycle will begin again after birth, everyone's period will return at a different time. The old-school myth that breastfeeding interferes with a cycle is not a blanket rule for everyone, but there is some truth to it. Most breastfeeding women will find they do not begin to menstruate in the first 3–6 months; this is called 'lactational amenorrhea'. However, the amount you are breastfeeding can impact this.

Most breastfeeding women find their period returns between 9 and 18 months postpartum. Once we begin weaning our little ones, our body will notice a decrease in the feeding demands and this can trigger our cycle to restart.

However, although 9–18 months is common, many mothers find their period returns earlier, whether breastfeeding or not. Some ladies might also find they experience a period-like bleed before 6 months, but then don't have another for a long time. This is because the initial bleed was a non-ovulatory period and the true menstrual cycle has not yet started.

In case you've been wondering this whole time about the old wives' tale that you don't need contraception until your period returns, or after you have finished breastfeeding, let me round up this chapter by busting that myth.

May I introduce you to my twins . . . Case in point.

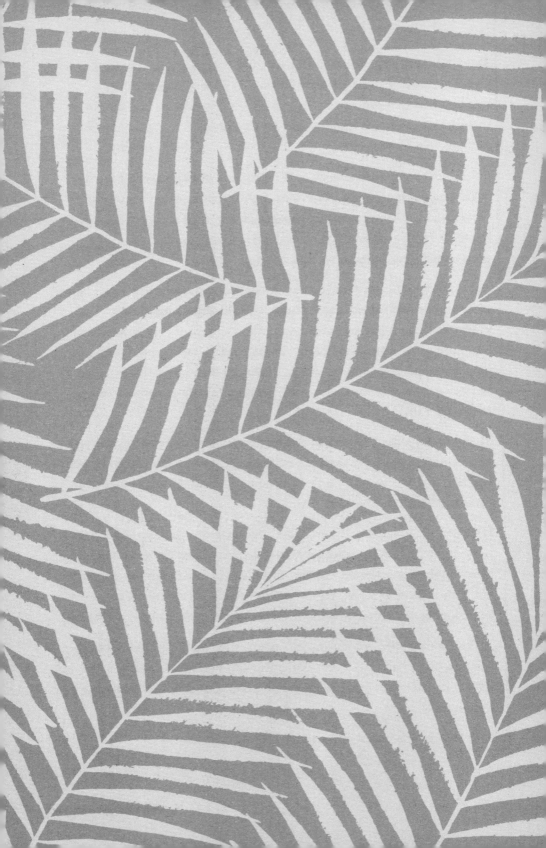

Prenatal nutrition

with Katie Shore

How humans view food has changed over the years.

I remember listening to a podcast with James Nestor, author of *Breathe*, in which he discussed the basic function of chewing. More and more foods are being puréed or turned into smoothies these days. In fact, there are even entire diet fads that promote supplementing solid foods with chemically processed, puréed alternatives.

The idea behind purées is that we'll need to chew less, meaning it's easier for our gut to digest the food and extract nutrients. But there are many other benefits from eating that are lost if we focus on a liquid diet. And these factors are hugely important to our overall health.

The simple act of chewing is one such example. How much we use our mouths when we eat will define the structure of our face. Even during the early years of weaning, chewing helps our face and neck muscles to develop. It can even dictate how our teeth sit and therefore how our face is shaped.

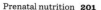

Of course the nutritional content of what we're eating is also of the utmost importance. We can't live off gobstoppers all day just because they work the mouth (if you don't remember these classic sweets, then just imagine a huge ball of sugar blown up to about the size of a tennis ball and you'll have the rough idea)!

We all know that a balanced diet is best, but how do our needs change during and after pregnancy? As I'm not a nutritional specialist myself, I knew that I needed to call on an expert to give you all of the wisdom you need. Fortunately I'm friends with just such a professional, fertility food specialist and mother, Katie Shore (@katielshore).

Pregnancy nutrition

Katie kicked off our conversation with a fact that surprised me. 'As beautiful and awe-inspiring as growing a baby can be, essentially, for our body, the foetus is like a parasite.'

Well that was a chipper start, I thought, people will love to read that about their babies! But Katie had a point: although it might not sound very nice, we can't escape the truth that, as soon as conception has taken place, a foetus is taking from our nutrition stores and energy levels, much as a parasite lives off its host. Okay, I promise to stop using the word parasite from now on, and only refer to babies as beautiful, snuggly love muffins!

❝WE ALL KNOW THAT A BALANCED DIET IS BEST, BUT HOW DO OUR NEEDS DURING AND AFTER PREGNANCY AFFECT WHAT THIS MEANS?❞

This dependency on our nutritional reservoir begins immediately after implantation. So our healthy nutritional habits should really be starting from around 3 months before the first trimester begins. Don't worry if you're already well into pregnancy and just reading this, it's never too late to make better food choices. Although eating healthily a few months before we conceive means that we can build up sufficient vitamin and mineral stores, so that there are already lots of nutrients for our baby to use right away, the truth is that whether you've been living off kale or crisps, your body will prioritise giving your baby what it needs. If you are lacking any nutrients, it's most likely you as the mother who will experience the deficiency.

Our gut health should always be high up on our priority list too, but particularly pre- and postnatally. We've already touched on how our gut health can affect our postnatal recovery and it's equally important for pregnancy. New research has shown that healthy gut bacteria and elements of a mother's gut microbiome are passed on to baby whilst still in utero.[21] 'We used to think babies were sterile in the womb,' Katie told me, 'but now we know that the health of our own gut during pregnancy will directly impact the foundations of our child's stomach flora.'

This connection between mum and baby lasts during pregnancy and beyond. 'Even postpartum, if a mother chooses to breastfeed, there are certain cells in the body that pinch healthy microbes from the mother's gut. These cells then travel to the nipple and are passed on to our baby via breastmilk. So it's never too late to start a healthy diet.'

Let's start by looking at nutrition from early pregnancy and then through the trimesters.

The first trimester

'The first trimester is all about initial development and laying healthy building blocks for your growing baby,' Katie told me. 'By twelve weeks' gestation your baby's major organs have formed: the brain, heart, lungs, kidneys, liver, arms and legs have all been established and the placenta is also fully developed. In these early days we want to make sure a mother has well-balanced blood sugar levels. This can help us to avoid gestational diabetes.'

How to balance your blood sugar

Blood sugar, also known as glucose, is what our body uses to break down and create energy. It is the main sugar found in the food we eat. It's not the only way our body can create energy, but maintaining good blood sugar levels helps our body deliver nutrients to our organs, muscles and the nervous system to help with everyday functions.

Despite the name 'sugar', this doesn't mean we need lots of sweets to hit the spot. Sugars are also found in carbohydrates, and the make-up of these types of sugars, called complex sugars, is much better for giving us long-lasting energy than the simple sugars found in sweets.

After food is broken down in our stomach, most substances are passed into the intestines. It's here that glucose and other vitamins, minerals, proteins and water are all absorbed into the body, whilst waste is excreted via the back passage.

Our endocrine system then kicks in via the pancreas to produce the hormone insulin, which our body uses to manage the levels of glucose in our body. It does this in two ways.

Ideally, if our blood sugar levels are balanced, the glucose is transported around the body and used as energy. But, if blood sugar levels are raised, the excess glucose is sent to the liver to be stored in a new form called glycogen. If our blood sugar levels are low, however, the pancreas can also produce another hormone called glucagon, which does the opposite of insulin and raises our blood sugar levels when needed. If the body needs more sugar in the blood, glucagon signals to the liver to turn glycogen back into glucose and release it back into our bloodstream. This is how our blood sugar levels stay balanced.

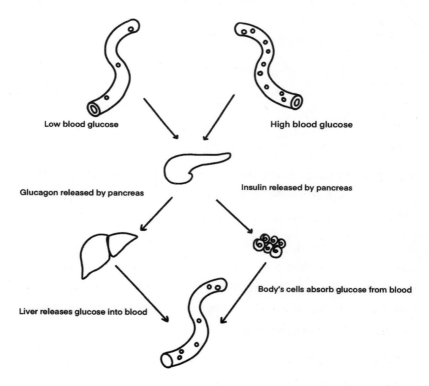

Low blood glucose

High blood glucose

Glucagon released by pancreas

Insulin released by pancreas

Body's cells absorb glucose from blood

Liver releases glucose into blood

Normal blood glucose levels

Constant high levels of blood sugar can be detrimental to our health and can develop into conditions like Type 1 and Type 2 diabetes. Type 1 diabetes happens when the body struggles to produce enough insulin to help break down and distribute the glucose, whereas Type 2 diabetes occurs when your pancreas can produce insulin just fine, but the cells in your body don't use it the way they should. This is known as insulin resistance.

When our cells don't know how to utilise the insulin, this confuses our body and at first our pancreas tries to make more insulin to get the glucose into our cells. Eventually it can't keep up with the demand it thinks we need and the glucose builds up in our blood.

During pregnancy, our placenta produces hormones which may make it difficult for our body to use insulin as it should. This puts us at an increased risk of developing insulin resistance, and if our body can't produce enough insulin to overcome it, this can cause glucose to build up in our blood and we may be diagnosed with gestational diabetes. Eating too much sugar or being too sedentary (not moving enough) can all increase our likelihood of gestational diabetes, particularly during pregnancy when insulin demands are already increased.

If left untreated, continued levels of high blood sugar could cause some health complications for mum and baby. However, once gestational diabetes has been diagnosed, it can be monitored and managed well. Our dietary choices can have a huge impact on the prevention and control of gestational diabetes.

When I asked exactly how we can manage our blood sugar during pregnancy, Katie talked to me a lot about The Rainbow Diet theory, which suggests eating foods of a variety of different colours and textures. 'We need many different fruits and vegetables to ensure that we have a good balance of all the vitamins and minerals we need,' Katie said. 'This will allow us to maintain healthy blood sugar levels alongside keeping our immune system on top form, our skin and bones healthy, whilst also supporting the development of our foetus.'

Although we shouldn't judge a book by its cover (even a cover as nice as the one on this book), when it comes to fruits and vegetables, appearance can tell us a lot. For example, not all apples are the same. Green apples usually contain higher levels of vitamins and fibre, whereas red apples are higher in anti-oxidants and sugar. The same is true for other fruits and vegetables too.

❛OUR DIETARY CHOICES CAN HAVE A HUGE IMPACT ON THE PREVENTION AND CONTROL OF GESTATIONAL DIABETES.❜

Taste the rainbow

Green: Dark greens like avocados, broccoli, asparagus, kiwis, spinach and beans are all examples of foods high in iron, vitamins K, C and E and folate, which help our babies' brain development as well as encouraging healthy skin, eyes and bones in both mum and baby.

Deep blue/purple: Blueberries, blackberries, black olives, aubergines, passion fruit, acai berries and purple grapes are full of antioxidants which can help a pregnant mama's immunity and prevent infections.

Red: Beets, strawberries, red apples, cherries, pomegranates and tomatoes aren't just pretty to look at, they are nutritious powerhouses too! Along with all the vitamins and minerals they provide, these foods also contain substances known as phytochemicals which help to control high blood pressure in pregnancy.

Yellow/orange: Pumpkins, carrots, oranges, sweetcorn, lemons and mangos are bright, beautiful and brilliant for our bellies. They are a fab source of folate to help baby's development and they also help sustain recommended levels of vitamin A. There are health warnings around not consuming too much vitamin A during pregnancy; however, Katie assured me 'the type of vitamin A that pregnant women need to avoid over-consuming is vitamin A from animal products such as liver. Eating too many carrots shouldn't be an issue for anyone!'

Pale/brown: Bananas, garlic, mushrooms, ginger and potatoes are all fab too. They promote healthy digestion and contain high levels of antioxidants.

As you can see, eating a variety of colours in our diet is beneficial. Now let's chat through some of the most important vitamins!

Vital vitamin D

'Vitamin D is an interesting one,' Katie said. 'Keeping adequate stores of vitamin D helps us maintain good gut health, and supports both our own and our baby's immune system. However, we also need enough levels of vitamin D in our body to absorb calcium.

There are certain vitamins that we must have in our body in order to absorb other minerals; we refer to them as "catalysts" and vitamin D is a catalyst for calcium. Calcium supports healthy bone development for our baby as well as kidney, heart and nervous-system function.'

We can get a lot of vitamin D from sunlight, but during pregnancy our demands are increased as our body must provide these vitamins and minerals for our baby as well as for ourselves. 'As recommended by the NHS, I'd recommend women take 10-microgram supplements of vitamin D (400IU) a day during pregnancy, and we can use food to boost our stores,' said Katie. 'Good sources of vitamin D include oily fish like salmon, red meat and egg yolks. There are also some cereals which have been fortified with extra levels of vitamin D and calcium.'

Iron

Iron is a mineral, used by the body to create a substance called haemoglobin. This is present in red blood cells and helps to carry and deliver oxygen to other parts of our body so that our cells can produce energy. Iron also helps to remove carbon dioxide from the body.

During pregnancy our blood volume is increased, and we need the additional iron in our blood to keep up with the higher levels of red blood cells.

Iron deficiency can be common in pregnancy: because our blood volume is so much higher, therefore the demand for iron increases too. If the body struggles to meet the demand for iron, we may be diagnosed with prenatal anaemia and prescribed iron tablets.

In the same way we need vitamin D to absorb calcium, we need vitamin C in order for our body to absorb iron. 'Simply squeezing some lemon juice onto our salad or drinking a drop after consuming iron-rich foods will help our body to absorb this mineral,' advised Katie.

Iron-rich foods include red meat, beans, nuts, beetroot, spinach, dried fruit and strawberries. Katie recommends strawberries because not only do they contain iron, but also high levels of vitamin C, making it easy for our body to digest both together. Other foods rich in vitamin C are citrus fruits, peppers, blackcurrants, broccoli, Brussels sprouts and potatoes.

Frolic with folate

Possibly the most talked about prenatal nutrient, folic acid tablets are recommended even before conception and are needed in quite high levels throughout pregnancy. But folic acid is actually a synthetic form of this nutrient, which in its natural form is known as folate. Consuming the natural version, by eating folate-rich foods can provide an added bonus to our prenatal health and our baby's development.

I remember consuming huge amounts of asparagus in early pregnancy because I wanted to boost my folate stores as much as possible. But what other foods, I asked Katie, can provide us with natural sources of folate? 'There are tons,' Katie began. 'Lots of your leafy green vegetables, as well as broccoli, Brussels sprouts, peas, kidney beans and lots of cereals which are fortified with folic acid.'

First trimester fish tales

'Fish oils are a controversial topic in pregnancy,' Katie admitted. 'We face a bit of a conundrum, because although we'd ideally get our nutrients from natural sources by consuming at least three portions of oily fish a week, unfortunately supermarket fish is often contaminated with heavy metals, which we want to avoid.'

These metals can find their way into marine life via current agriculture and mining methods, which can lead to significant amounts of heavy metals in the marine ecosystems. 'This doesn't mean we shouldn't eat any fish at all though,' Katie confirmed. 'Fish oil is highly recommended to support brain, eye and nerve development for our babies in utero. Ideally we should be including one or two portions of oily fish like salmon, trout, mackerel or herring per week, and use a good-quality fish oil supplement alongside for additional support.'

Healthy hydration

A person's body weight when not pregnant is already made up of between 55 and 65 per cent water, making this the most common element in the body!

Hydration is a balancing act. On one side is dehydration and on the other over-hydration. We want to straddle the line of not consuming too many liquids, which could mean our salt levels become diluted, but also not under-consuming liquids, which leads to dehydration.

During pregnancy, our body needs extra stores of water to support the increased blood volume, amniotic fluid and other energy requirements like preparing for breastfeeding. The need for more water increases as the trimesters progress.

Research suggests that we need about 1:1.5 ml of water per calorie. Don't panic, this doesn't involve complex maths – and that's coming from someone who was in set D in secondary school. An average daily diet is about 2,000 calories, so that would equate to about 2,000–3,000ml of water. That's about eight medium-sized glasses of water per day.

In the second trimester the Royal College of Obstetrics and Gynaecologists (RCOG) recommends an extra 340 calories a day, adding an extra 340–510ml, or between one and one-and-a-half extra glasses of water per day.

During the third trimester this increases again, but only by about 100 calories, which means we should be up to ten glasses of water a day.

Water doesn't just have to come in the form of a drink though. Different foods have different water contents. Some foods, like cucumbers, strawberries, melon, lettuce and yogurts have a high water content and can help to keep us hydrated.

If you're now wondering how on Earth to measure how many millilitres of water are in a yogurt, let me stop you right there. Our body isn't relying on our maths skills to stay hydrated. It gives us plenty of signs that it's lacking in fluids, many of which occur long before we feel thirsty. These include dry mouth or lips, feeling tired, infrequent urination, dark-coloured or strong-smelling urine and dry eyes.

Anything that encourages our body to excrete excess water or that demands extra fluids can increase our likelihood of dehydration, like vomiting, diarrhoea, consuming alcohol or caffeine, exercise, sweating and having a temperature.

Managing morning sickness

Oh how I wish I'd had this information when I was pregnant! 'Balancing your blood sugar is so important for women struggling with morning sickness because when you feel nauseous, an extreme sugar high and the subsequent low is only going to make you feel worse,' Katie explained. 'Small, frequent meals or lots of little snacks will help you sustain a good level of blood sugar; you don't need to force down three big meals if you're not up to it. Even having snacks by your bed to keep your levels up during the night or as soon as you wake up can help.'

Let's get straight to the facts on this one. What snacks can actually help us combat morning sickness? I really hope one of these suggestions works for you.

Ginger

You hear a lot about ginger helping to ease morning sickness, but personally I got fed up with people suggesting it because it didn't seem to work for me. However, I didn't realise that you need to give it a few days to kick in, so maybe this is where I went wrong. I read a medical paper which suggested that taking ginger capsules containing 250mg of ginger, four times a day, might be effective, or that a quarter teaspoon of grated raw ginger root in a cup of boiling water can be equally helpful.[22] Research found that a large percentage of women who consumed 1,000mg of ginger daily from early pregnancy experienced significantly less nausea and fewer vomiting episodes than those who took a placebo.[23]

Some evidence suggests that ginger should not be consumed too close to labour as this may increase the risk of bleeding. But there is no research that suggests ginger has any negative effect on pregnancy early on for mum or baby. Nonetheless, pregnant women with a history of miscarriage, vaginal bleed or blood clotting should consult a medical professional before trying any ginger products.

B vitamins

I tried vitamin B tablets to ease my morning sickness as well (I mean, I tried pretty much everything!). Although, again, no one told me these should be taken regularly for best results. Apparently we should be taking the supplement at least three times a day to have an effect.

Research suggests that it's specifically vitamin B6 that can have a positive impact on nausea. A typical dose is between 10–25mg, three times a day.

Sour foods

'Tart tastes can be a great way to reduce nausea. But it comes down to your cravings. Some love the idea, whilst others can't even bear the thought,' Katie told me. 'Some of my favourite sour sensations in pregnancy were citrus fruits, like oranges, lemons and limes, which can be eaten raw or added to water for a refreshing drink. Other sour flavours include bitter leaves like endives, peppery rocket and radicchio or olives and pickles.'

Cold foods

As much as I like to shatter stereotypes, you know that clichéd image of a pregnant woman crunching ice chips all day? Well, that was me! Ice chips and fizzy water were never far from my grasp.

'Cold foods often smell less pungent and take less time to prepare,' Katie shared. 'One of my favourite remedies for pregnancy is frozen smoothie ice-cubes. You can make them by blending together your favourite fruits or vegetables with some water, juice or almond milk and freezing them in an ice tray. This allows you to get in sufficient nutrients, whilst also reducing nausea with the cold sensation.'

Other cold foods which might help nausea include: frozen grapes or pomegranates, smoothies, ice lollies or chilled carbonated (fizzy) water.

Salty foods

'Unless you've been clinically diagnosed with high blood pressure, salty foods like miso soup can help to ease nausea and support our adrenal glands,' Katie said.

I did a little more digging into these benefits and it turns out that our adrenal glands are small glands found on top of our kidneys that help to produce hormones that support blood pressure control within our body. Too much salt isn't good, as this can make it difficult for our kidneys to remove excess water from our bloodstream, leading to high blood pressure. But we don't want to dip below a certain level of salt either. This can cause adrenal fatigue and our kidneys may start to hold on to sodium rather than functioning as they should.

During pregnancy, with the increased level of blood volume in our body, our need for more sodium (salt) increases as well. We need to keep our water and salt levels balanced.

The honest truth

Whilst all the above tips are great and yes, we want to make sure that our nutrition is as healthy as possible, sometimes, we've just got to eat what we can!

I've been there: weeks on end of nothing but sugary, dry cereal, bread and salty crisps with not a vegetable in sight! Ladies, we sometimes just have to embrace survival mode. I'm not sure all nutritionists would agree, but if you find you just fancy a packet of salt and vinegar crisps and naught else, you have my full support!

There are of course some cases where morning sickness does need further advice from medical professionals. If you feel overwhelmed by the nausea make sure to mention this to you midwife or GP and discuss additional support.

TART TASTES CAN BE A GREAT WAY TO REDUCE NAUSEA. BUT IT COMES DOWN TO YOUR CRAVINGS. SOME LOVE THE IDEA, WHILST OTHERS CAN'T EVEN BEAR THE THOUGHT.

The second trimester

I already told you the second trimester is one of my favourites in terms of how our energy levels feel. For our baby it means further development and growth, and our nutritional choices play a part in supporting this. Although many of your baby's vital organs are already formed by the start of the second trimester, muscles and bones continue to develop, and hair, eyelashes and eyebrows begin to grow. Your baby will also start to hear sounds like your heartbeat by around 18 weeks and sensory neurones begin to function, like taste, touch and hearing.

Fascinating stuff, isn't it?

So what are the top nutritional tips we need to be aware of? Along with all of the vitamins and minerals from the first trimester Katie highly recommends taking a multivitamin, but cautions that we do want to be careful which one we choose.

Vital vs misleading multivitamins

According to Katie, not all pregnancy multivitamins are the same, despite what the branding might have you believe, as some of the more well-known brands have lots of additional fillers or excipients in them.

An excipient is a substance that is included in some pharmaceutical medications, not for their therapeutic action but to support the manufacturing process. 'They're not dangerous in such low dosages,' Katie said. 'However they can make it more challenging for your gut to break down the tablet and extract the vitamins, which can often delay the effectiveness of the product reaching your system.'

In addition to a multivitamin, Katie encourages women to take a daily vitamin D tablet and a probiotic, specifically for pregnancy and breastfeeding.

Probiotics are a combination of live bacteria already found in the human body. We all have 'good' bacteria and 'bad' bacteria. Probiotic supplements are full of the good bacteria our body needs, which can help us to fight off other infections and keep our body working well. Research on the full effect of probiotics is in its early days, but alongside keeping our gut healthy, the studies that have been done have shown some intriguing suggestions.

Some studies suggest that taking regular probiotics in pregnancy to support a diverse bacterial gut formation can protect us against certain pregnancy complications, including pre-term labour.[24]

B-aware

B vitamins continue to be essential in the second trimester. 'B vitamins are water soluble,' Katie explained, 'which means that our body doesn't hold on to them. Whatever we don't use is excreted in our waste. This is why we need to make sure that they are a part of our everyday diet. Along with the B vitamin supplement that we're taking, we can consume foods like leafy green vegetables, red meat, chicken and dairy to get a higher level of this vitamin. For those following a vegan diet, nutritional yeast is a fantastic option. As always though, we should always consult our GP before taking anything new in pregnancy.'

Consider choline

Nope, I hadn't heard of this either, but according to Katie, choline is a micronutrient that's been gaining popularity since the start of the century.

'Similar to folate, choline helps with baby's neural tubes and brain development,' Katie told me. 'Eggs are a fantastic bio-available source and it's also in beans, peas, lentils and pulses, like sunflower seeds and kidney beans, as well as cauliflower and broccoli.'

The third trimester

In the third trimester our body has two main focuses: the first is preparing our body for labour and the second is increasing the fat stores, muscles and bones of our baby.

'There's a misconception that we need to be eating for two at this stage,' Katie said, 'but it's a complete myth. We only want to increase our calorie intake by about 300–500 calories, or a maximum of 900–1,350 if carrying twins or multiples.'

Target tryptophan

Katie explained that tryptophan is an amino acid, which means it's a compound found in protein, such as poultry. 'It's important that we consume this as part of our diet because it can't be produced in the body, so food is our only way of reaping the benefits! It helps our body with various processes like building muscle and regulating immune functions and it encourages quality sleep.'

But this is just one way we can prepare for labour. Labour is effectively an endurance exercise so we want to prep our body accordingly.

Labour meal prep

'It's tempting for the last few weeks of pregnancy to become "party weeks" where nutrition is concerned,' Katie told me. 'Everyone takes on a "YOLO" attitude and indulges in unhealthy foods as a way to celebrate impending parenthood. But I'd seriously suggest getting some nutrients in there too, because unhealthy foods mean you'll be left depleted quickly after eating.' When you get those nesting urges in the final few weeks, start prepping your labour snacks! Iron-rich foods are also important as are lots of quality protein and carbohydrates. 'Every macro- and micronutrient plays its role,' said Katie. 'Fats are important to prepare for breastmilk production. Protein helps to build muscle and aids an efficient recovery. Carbohydrates form the start of our energy system and fibre encourages healthy digestion. All of this is crucial during and after labour.'

Longevity foods for labour

If we want to keep high energy levels throughout labour, we need to get to grips with balancing our blood sugar levels. 'It's all well and good enjoying chocolate in the excitement, and it will give you an instant high, but if we want energy for the long haul, we really need to indulge in foods that will keep our energy up long term. Chocolates and other sweet treats are a bit of a false economy,' Katie said. 'They give you an instant high, but in the long run they will only leave you feeling run down.

'Fluid intake is also important, but I'd highly recommend avoiding sugary energy drinks because again they're usually short-term fuel. Coconut water is great, as it's full of electrolytes which help to stabilise our blood pressure.'

Another great recipe Katie shared with me was the 'Orange Zinger', which is a super quick and simple concoction of 100ml coconut water combined with 100ml of orange juice and a pinch of salt, to help replenish hydration and also vitamins and minerals.

The concept of eating during labour was new to me. I'd never eaten in labour because epidurals and spinals meant a nil-by-mouth policy, but many women do continue to eat snacks during this time, whether at home, in the water, or with a mobile labour.

'There are tons of quick, energy-boosting snacks that are also good to support your body in labour and recovery,' Katie told me. 'We want "grab-and-go" snacks, like veg sticks, hummus and cheese. If you've been able to pre-prepare them, frittatas are great to keep in the fridge and eat during labour too.'

'Bananas are a wonder food! They will give you a quick energy hit that also sustains you and gives you a nutritional boost. Dried fruits and nuts are also great for healthy fats and fibre. There's no one food to choose. What's most important is that we make conscious choices with our nutrition overall.'

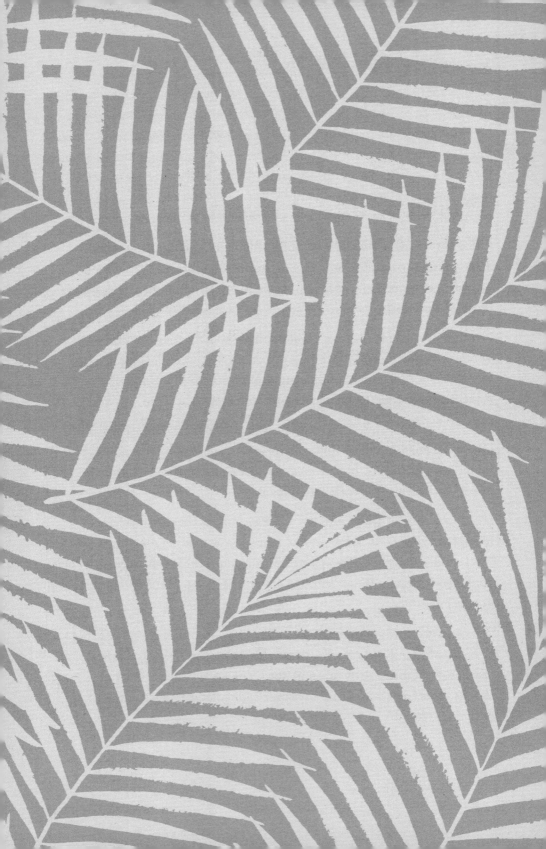

Postnatal nutrition

with Katie Shore and Catherine Rabess

In this chapter we start with the days immediately after labour and continue with nutritional advice that can support you throughout your entire first year. I should say that despite the advice in this chapter, sometimes when chaotic moments of mum-life hit, in my opinion just making sure you consume anything is great, even if that is a slice of bread and a coffee.

As you can already tell from that advice I just shared, even those of us who know what we should be doing don't always stick to it! But it goes without saying that we want to try our best to consume the right foods and here's the inside scoop on what that is!

First foods

If you're anything like me you'll want to celebrate your baby's arrival with a big slice of cake, followed by your favourite chocolate, sweets, fizzy drink and ice cream! 'Give me what tastes good,' I declared, 'because I deserve it!!'

That last bit of the mentality is where the contradiction lies. I wanted to treat my body to a slice of cake, but really it's not a treat at all, it's just more hard work for a body already drained by labour.

I don't think anyone needs a lecture from me to know that cake and sweets aren't the best idea nutritionally speaking. The energy demands of labour are immense and, although wanting to celebrate is fine, what our body also needs is quality fuel to repair and recover.

'If you want that celebration aspect and the healthy food just isn't hitting the spot, dark chocolate with over 70 per cent cocoa can give us some great health benefits alongside the desired sugar hit,' Katie recommended. One of those good things dark chocolate can provide us with is magnesium. 'Honestly,' Katie told me, 'it's such an underrated micronutrient.'

Marvellous magnesium

Magnesium is a super nutrient, especially for us new mums as it's used in every cell of our body. It helps convert food into energy, as well as regulating our nervous system, whilst helping our body to create new proteins, which are the building blocks for our muscles, bones, skin and more.

Alongside keeping our body functions efficient, magnesium can also help to improve our sleep, help us feel relaxed, and, when needed, sustain our energy. 'I know, it sounds like an oxymoron,' Katie said when I looked at her in disbelief. 'It sounds strange to suggest that magnesium can play a role in increasing our energy or encourage rest and sleep when needed, but it can. In short, magnesium connects to so many different cells throughout our system that there can be various ripple effects, depending on the function our body is trying to achieve.

'Magnesium is essential for an extraordinary number of functions in the body,' Katie said. 'And being even a little bit deficient can leave your energy levels low and sleep pattern in disarray.'

Another one of its seemingly endless functions is helping our muscles to contract and, by assisting with the formation of certain proteins, it also helps our body grow, develop and function in multiple ways.

Foods that are high in magnesium include avocados; nuts such as almonds, cashews and Brazil nuts; legumes; tofu; flaxseeds; pumpkin seeds; chia seeds; whole grains like wheat, oats and barley; bananas; and – I'm happy to confirm – dark chocolate!

Fire-lighting foods

'All the food choices we make should support three key functions,' Katie told me. 'Number one: recharging our energy stores; two: repairing our muscles and other body tissues; and three: supporting a smooth and easy digestion.'

There are tons of foods we can eat to give us energy, but it's the long-lasting endurance ones that we need. 'It's useful to imagine our energy like a fire,' Katie said. 'High-sugar foods would be the equivalent of adding some tissue paper to the fire. It might light quickly and create a flame but it burns away almost as fast, leaving you with nothing. Good-quality foods on the other hand are like adding a chunky log to your fire; it might be slower to take but once lit, it will burn for much longer.'

I liked the idea of looking at nutrition as a fire and as I felt my tummy rumble and knew I needed to stoke the embers myself, I wanted to know what foods fell into which category and which would be most accessible for women immediately after birth.

Tissue paper foods	Log burners
Chocolate	Nut butters
Fizzy drinks	Tahini
Sweets	Oats
	Protein balls
	Full-fat yogurts
	Berries
	Falafel
	Hummus
	Eggs
	Guacamole

'THE INTERESTING THING ABOUT PROTEIN IS THAT WE NEED TO EAT A DIVERSE RANGE OF FOODS TO GET A GOOD AND VARIED AMOUNT. THERE ISN'T JUST ONE WAY OF MAKING PROTEIN IN THE BODY AND WE NEED ALL FORMS.'

Morsels for muscular repair

With energy ticked off the list it's time to turn our attention to foods that support muscular repair, and that's primarily protein, often referred to as 'the building blocks of life'.

Katie told me, 'When you're pregnant, your protein requirement increases with each trimester because your body needs to grow and stretch. Postpartum, to one degree or another, your body has gone through a form of trauma and, no matter how you gave birth, there is healing that needs to be done. Protein can help us do it!'

The interesting thing about protein is that we need to eat a diverse range of foods to get a good and varied amount. There isn't just one way of making protein in the body and we need all forms.

When I first learned about proteins, it was almost like when I first learnt about the universe at school. I was left awestruck. Like space, at first glance we see our planet but then we learn about the solar system, the stars, galaxies and then infinite eternity... Mind blown!

I felt similarly about proteins, although I do have a tendency to get carried away with things so let's see if you feel the same or not...

Scientists believe that there are seven main groups that a protein can fall under. These categories are antibodies, contractile proteins, enzymes, hormonal proteins, structural proteins, storage proteins and transport proteins. This gives you an insight into how important their role is. But, within these seven groups, scientists estimate that there could be tens of thousands of protein structures in total. One medical document I read proposed that numbers could fall 'between 10,000 and several billion different protein species'.[25]

I told you, mind blown!

But let's zoom back in and keep things simple.

If we're looking at just one protein, it is made up of a chain of smaller compounds called amino acids. If you imagine a string of pearls on a necklace, each individual pearl is an amino acid and the entire chain then becomes a protein. There are twenty amino acids in total. This is why there are so many variables in how a protein can be formed. The combination of amino acids can change.

Nine of these amino acids are known as 'essential' amino acids, and that's because they cannot be made in our body; we have to eat them in order for our body to be able to use them!

'One of the most important proteins for repair and recovery is collagen,' Katie told me. Unfortunately, the compounds of natural collagen can only be found in animal products so for people following a plant-based diet, it can be tricky to consume. 'There are some good quality synthetic-based collagen powders available on the market for anyone following a plant-based diet,' Katie confirmed. 'It might not be as good as the natural source but it's still a fab support for muscular repair.'

Collagen from meat is the best to help our body with structural and muscular repair. 'This is found in high levels in the gelatinous substances from meat,' Katie said. 'Those thick, jelly-like blobs you find in some home-made soups and sauces are the gelatin from the meat. This is where we'll find high levels of collagen. Bone broths are a great source for this as collagen comes from the sinew and bones of meat, where there is a high concentration of gelatin.' Katie went on to add that we can also find collagen in fish, 'and this type of collagen is brilliant for supporting skin and hair regrowth and composition.' The added benefit from fish is that we also get the support of Omega 3 and the essential fatty acids.

The digestion question

No matter how you've given birth, many mothers are probably aware of the pressures surrounding that first postpartum poop. Immediately after delivery the idea of straining in the pelvic floor area can be nerve-wracking. But sometimes being able to pass a stool can be the difference between you going home and being asked to stay in hospital an extra night.

Eating foods to ease our digestion means we won't need to strain in order to pass a motion, lowering the risk of haemorrhoids, which can become uncomfortable and irritating to say the least. Plus, having a smooth digestive tract will help to alleviate any pressure that could build up behind the incision after a caesarean section.

Soups, smoothies, stews, casseroles and broths are all a good choice, as are foods that contain quality fibre! Foods that are high in fibre include fruits – like apples, pears and raspberries – and vegetables – like avocados, carrots, broccoli and Brussels sprouts. Lentils, beans and oats also contain high levels of fibre.

Katie's words reminded me of another conversation I'd had recently with a good friend of mine, Catherine Rabess (@caffdietitian) who specialises in gut health. Catherine also talked about fibre. 'Foods rich in prebiotics are dietary fibres which can help to feed our beneficial gut microbes.'

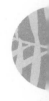

As a total novice to *prebiotics* and *probiotics*, I needed a little more explanation about what exactly they were. 'Probiotics are live bacteria and yeasts added to food or that come in supplement form. They help to restore the beneficial bacteria in the gut, and prebiotics are effectively the food for this bacteria,' said Catherine. 'With the dramatic changes in hormones during the pre- and postnatal period, and with a significant number of hormones being produced in the gut (for example, 90 per cent of serotonin), it's important to keep our gut microbiome thriving so that they can support our growing baby and other pre- and postnatal body functions.'

Foods high in prebiotics include apples, artichokes, asparagus, onions, garlic, leeks, amaranth, barley, cashews, freekeh, pistachios, rye, spelt, legumes (beans, chick peas, gungo peas, etc.), chamomile tea, dandelion tea, apricots, dates, peaches, pears, plums, beetroot, Brussels sprouts, fennel, okra, almonds, hazelnuts, seeds, edamame beans, dried mango/figs, nectarines, grapefruit, kiwi fruit and prunes. All these foods are quality prebiotics, supporting our healthy gut bacteria.

'Probiotics can be classed as the good, or friendly, bacteria,' Catherine continued. 'They can be found in foods with added live cultures, including natural live yoghurt, aged hard cheese, kombucha, miso, sauerkraut and kefir. In addition, many plants contain polyphenols, which are plant chemicals rich in antioxidants and can help to prevent and reverse damage to our cells. These are found in large amounts in berries, spices and herbs such as cloves, oregano, mint, nuts, flaxseeds, artichokes, onions, olives, even dark chocolate as long as it is more than 75 per cent solids.'

Breastfeeding bites

So we've covered most of the immediate postnatal period. What foods you choose are down to you, and don't worry if a bar of chocolate accidentally hops out of your bag and into your mouth, it's happened to all of us! Maybe just try to include one of two other nutrients as well to balance out the effect.

There's one more area of motherhood, though, where nutrition plays a big part and that's with breastfeeding. Whether or not breastfeeding is the right choice for you and your baby is, of course, completely down to you. No one should feel judged for their choice of feeding, and, as a mother who has breastfed, bottle-fed and used a combination, I know that each approach has its benefits. If you do choose to breastfeed, here are some facts to mull over, and information about nutrients to support your supply.

'Oats are like breastmilk's best friend,' Katie told me. 'They contain high levels of iron which helps to support milk production; however, there is a substance that is even more important than this, and that's water! Staying hydrated is a top priority for breastfeeding women.'

Breastmilk is 88 per cent water. It's suggested that breastfeeding women try to have at least sixteen 8-ounce cups of water a day. That might sound like a lot but, actually, you will feel a natural thirst that will inspire you to drink more anyway. 'The water doesn't need to just come from drinks,' Katie added. 'Herbal teas can be a great way to stay hydrated and benefit from some extra nutrients. Fennel and fenugreek seeds, for example, are thought to deliver great breastfeeding benefits and some women have found it supports supply as well.'

Fennel seeds have another benefit, that might draw us to them even more as mothers. 'Not only are they great for breastfeeding, but the effect of this seed is said to settle an uneasy tummy, and it can pass through our breastmilk to baby and help to settle any colic distress for windy babies.'

Along with oats and water, Katie mentioned brewer's yeast to support breastfeeding and overall postnatal health. 'Similar to nutritional yeast, which we mentioned for prenatal nutrition, brewer's yeast is not an active yeast, so it won't expand or ferment in your belly. We can use this just as a supplement and add it to any recipes for a nutritional boost. It works really well in smoothies or lactation cookies.'

If you're wondering what exactly a lactation cookie is, this and many more recipes can be found at **StrongLikeMum.com**, easily accessed using the QR code below.

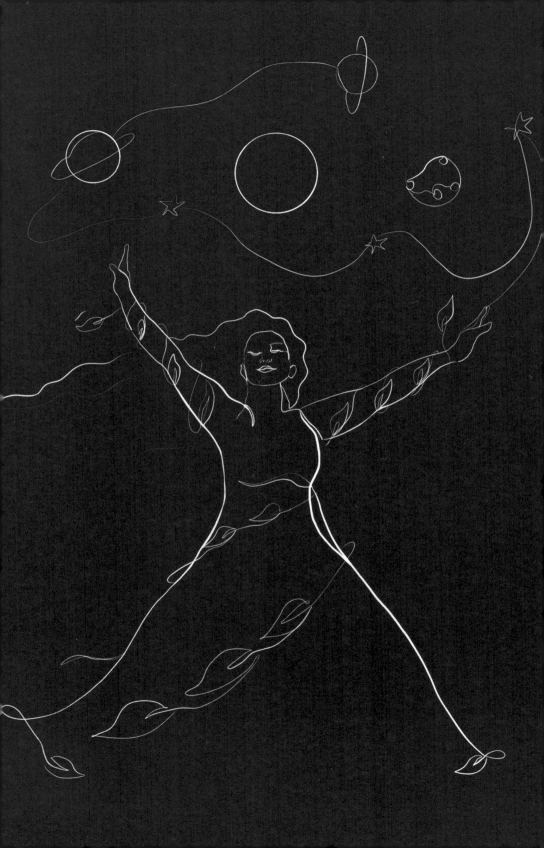

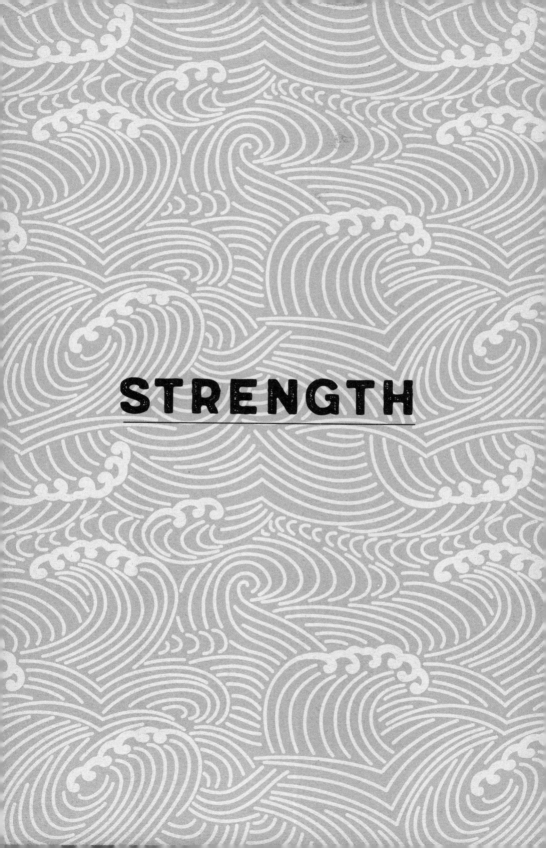

STRENGTH

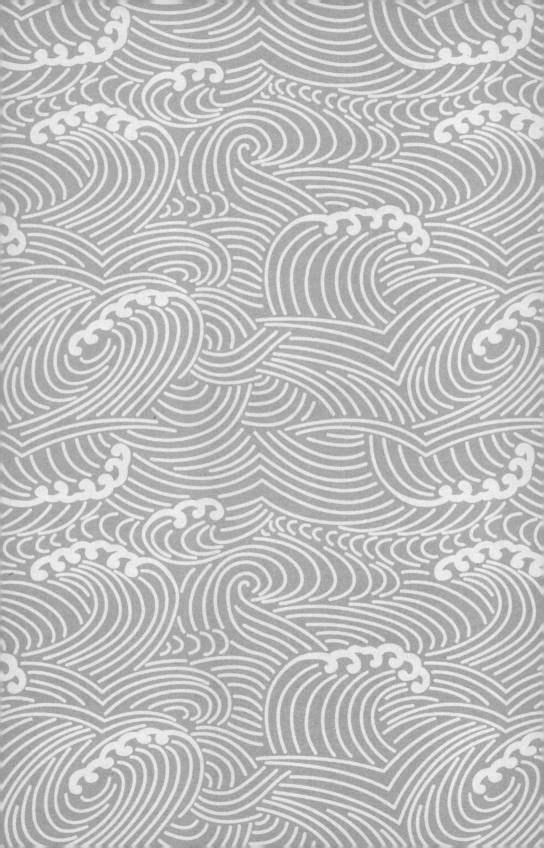

Movements to support motherhood

As a mother, I'm always amazed that there aren't clearer guidelines on how to progress exercises safely in the postnatal period. This lack of information is a failing on the part of the fitness industry for all women. No mother should be made to feel like her recovery is out of her control or be unsure of how to manage her own body.

I remember leaving hospital after the birth of my first son and being handed an A4 piece of paper which gave me a description of how to perform a Kegel exercise, some breastfeeding tips and suggestions on contraception. Charming!

It almost feels as though things are lined up for mothers to recover to a certain extent, reaching *acceptable* levels of health but never encouraging women to strive for *optimal* recovery.

In reality we should be supporting women to achieve their best possible health as mothers. Even if you consider yourself a beginner before pregnancy, we can use the postnatal stage as an opportunity to strip things back to basics and build a strong and stable body from the core outwards, moving forwards with more mobility, strength and confidence than ever before.

I say, let's aim to thrive as opposed to only survive.

How do you know when you're ready to progress?

It might sound daunting but, actually, progressing pre- and postnatal exercise is fairly simple. So far in this book we've rehabilitated our core, realigned our posture and worked on laying accurate core foundations. To move things onwards, half the battle is learning to read our body's signals correctly. It's constantly talking to us. We just need to learn how to listen to what it's saying.

I touched on some red flags in Chapter 5 that can be good indicators for when a movement is too challenging, and in the same way we can use markers that let us know we're ready to move on to a higher level of fitness. Let's call them green flags for the purpose of this chapter.

As always, if you have any reservations about progressing your exercise check in with your GP or a postnatal exercise expert and explain your concerns. Also, as outlined in the red flags, if you ever feel any pain, suffer unusual bleeding or feel faint or dizzy, stop, rest and consult a medical professional.

❝ TO MOVE THINGS ONWARDS, HALF THE BATTLE IS LEARNING TO READ OUR BODY'S SIGNALS CORRECTLY. ❞

Green flags

1 Complete core recovery

Before progressing our exercise programme, we want to be sure that we have rehabilitated our core. We've covered this in previous chapters so should now have a good level of function; however, for women with prolonged diastasis recti, where a gap under 2cm persists after 16–20 weeks postpartum, there are some specific exercises we can do to assist the healing process.

These exercises will encourage our core to strengthen steadily and safely so that we can create a 'functioning' diastasis, meaning we've achieved a strong support network of surrounding muscles, like our transverse abdominis and pelvic floor. If you notice a gap larger than 2cm wide, please speak with a medical professional about further investigation.

Along with assisting diastasis recti recovery, the following exercises and the lying pelvic tilt exercise in Chapter 10 are useful for rehabilitating a weakened pelvic floor, which could potentially cause urinary incontinence.

Urinary incontinence will affect around a third of women at some stage during the first year postpartum. However, although this is fairly common, it should in no way be something women settle for as their 'new normal'. Exercise can help to improve these symptoms. Should incontinence persist, have confidence in reaching out to your GP and asking for further investigation. More information on managing incontinence can be found on page 341.

Core recovery exercises

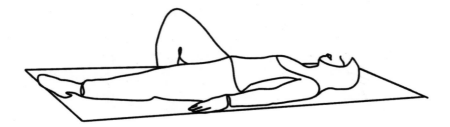

Exercise A: Heel slides

● Lie on the floor with your knees bent so that the soles of your feet are flat on the floor, hip-width apart.

● Your spine should be neutral and your arms relaxed at your sides.

● Inhale to prepare, and as you exhale, slowly release one leg, sliding it along the floor until it is fully extended, whilst drawing up your pelvic floor.

● Inhale and slide the extended leg back in towards you until it has reached the start position, with the sole of your foot back on the floor.

● Repeat on the other side.

● Your back should remain in its neutral position throughout this exercise.

● Repeat for 10–20 reps each side.

● Once you can comfortably perform 20 slides on each leg you may be ready to progress to the next exercise.

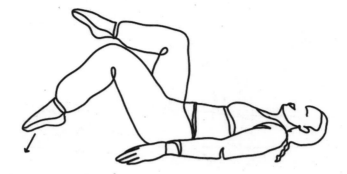

Exercise B: Toe taps

● Begin by lying flat on your back. Bring your legs up to a tabletop position, so that your knees are directly over your hips.

● Inhale to prepare, and as you exhale, keeping your knees bent, lower your right foot down towards the floor, tapping your toes on the ground. Simultaneously draw up your pelvic floor and focus on maintaining stable pelvic alignment.

● Be careful not to arch your back as your leg is lowered.

● Inhale as you bring your leg back up to the tabletop position.

● Repeat on the other side.

● Once you can comfortably perform 10 reps on each leg for 3 sets, you can progress to the next exercise.

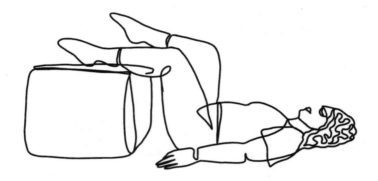

Exercise C: Elevated single leg lift

● Lie on your back with your calves supported on a chair, sofa or exercise bench. Your hips and knees should be at a 90-degree angle.

● Inhale to prepare, and as you exhale, draw up your pelvic floor and lift your right leg off the chair by about one inch.

● Hold for a count of eight.

● Inhale and lower your leg back onto your supporting platform.

● If you can comfortably perform this exercise for 10 reps each side you could be ready to try the progression.

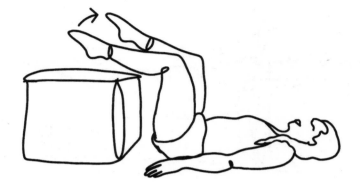

Progression: Double leg lift

● To progress this exercise, begin in the same position, lying on your back with your calves supported on a platform and your hips and knees bent to a 90-degree angle.

● Inhale, and as you exhale, engage your pelvic floor and lift your right leg off the platform, followed immediately by your left leg, which should lift off the platform to align with your right leg.

● Hold both legs off the chair for a count of eight.

● Inhale and release your right leg back onto the platform, followed immediately by your left leg.

● If you experience any back pain or feel your lower back arching as you lift your legs off, stop and modify the exercise back to a single leg raise only. There should be no doming or bulging of your abdominal muscles.

● Repeat for 10 reps.

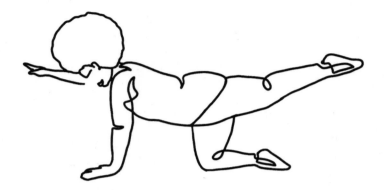

Exercise D: Bird-dog

● Begin in the four-point kneeling position, on your hands and knees with your hands shoulder-width apart and your knees directly under your hips, hip-width apart.

● Make sure your spine and head are in a neutral position.

● Inhale and as you exhale, extend your right arm and your left leg off the floor, whilst maintaining a stable pelvis and keeping your spine in neutral. Your arm should be extended straight out in front of you as your leg extends backwards.

● Hold for a count of 8. Inhale and lower both your right arm and left leg back to the start position.

● Exhale and perform this exercise on the other side, extending your left arm and right leg out, whilst drawing up your pelvic floor.

● Inhale and return to the start position.

● Perform 10 reps on each side.

A diastasis recti gap that remains over 2cm wide by the time we reach 16–20 weeks postpartum might benefit from further investigation by your medical team.

If we can perform these exercises whilst maintaining good form and without experiencing any back pain or clenching of our jaw or feet, it's a good sign that we're ready to progress our exercises to the next level.

2 Technique and pelvic stability

Alongside the exercises we've just covered, before progressing our workouts we should be able to perform movements with a stable and controlled pelvis. This means that we should be able to achieve good control of our glutes and deep core muscles, and perform movements without tilting to one side, gripping our toes or wobbling too much and falling off centre. In short, we have to be able to maintain good technique during movement before we move on to what's next.

A good way to test our pelvic stability is with the following exercises.

Single leg-hold stability test

● Stand tall with your feet hip-width apart, arms relaxed by your sides.

● Inhale and take a step forwards with your right foot, bringing your left hand forwards straight in front of you, in line with your right knee (image A).

● Bend your knees slightly, and as you exhale, push off your front foot, shifting your weight to balance on your left leg, bringing your left arm up overhead for balance (image B).

● Simultaneously draw up your pelvic floor.

● Hold for a count of five if possible.

● Inhale and return to the start position.

● Exhale and repeat on the other side.

● Repeat for 8 repetitions each side.

Performing this exercise in front of a mirror can help us to assess whether we have good core stability.

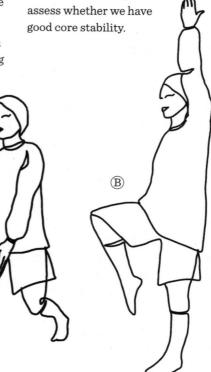

The next exercise was recommended to me by Grace Hurry (@gracehurrypilates), who shared the postnatal back extension exercise in Chapter 12. 'As a pilates practitioner and now instructor, I didn't truly realise the value of pilates until I found myself rehabilitating after a caesarean section,' Grace said, when I contacted her in regard to my own caesarean recovery. 'Establishing pelvic stability is important for all postnatal women, no matter what type of delivery they've experienced, as long as they have been cleared for exercise and have suffered no further medical complications. This hip-opening exercise helps to restore pelvic stability and engage the deep abdominals.'

'ESTABLISHING PELVIC STABILITY IS IMPORTANT FOR ALL POSTNATAL WOMEN, NO MATTER WHAT TYPE OF DELIVERY THEY'VE EXPERIENCED.'

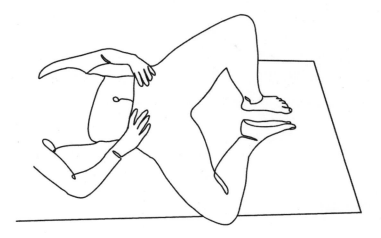

Hip opening and stability

● Begin by lying back on the floor, with your knees bent, soles of your feet flat to the floor and feet placed fist-distance apart.

● Rest your hands on your hips with your thumbs relaxed across your sides and fingers pointing towards your pubic bone.

● Inhale and open one knee out to the side whilst keeping the other leg very still. Focus on keeping the pelvis stable and the hip bones level.

● Exhale and return the open knee to the centre start position.

● Inhale and repeat on the other side.

● Continue in this way, slowly and with control. Repeat for 10 reps each side.

3 Easy reps

Coming up we have four circuits that are split into stages of progression. As well as the technical advice we've already looked at, we'll know when we're ready to move on to the next stage if we can complete the first workout easily. This might sound wishy-washy but if you find that you can complete all the sets and repetitions with bags of energy to spare it might be time to start progressing your workouts to the next level. To know that you are getting good benefits from a workout, you should begin to notice a tension or heaviness building in the muscle that is being worked about halfway through a set. This indicates that it's a good level for you to continue with for the moment. If you can complete your reps without feeling the work, you're most likely ready to move on.

4 RPE scale

When it comes to upping the intensity of our cardio exercises, RPE has been used in the fitness industry for years to help trainers and clients communicate how hard an exercise feels, and it's a fab way for us to keep in touch with our own progress as well.

RPE stands for Rate of Perceived Exertion and it's all about how hard we feel our body is working based on physical sensations, like sweating, heart rate, increased breathing rate, etc.

There are various versions out there, but for the sake of simplicity let's stick to the modified RPE scale that works from 0–10. This modified version is based mostly on breathlessness but we should always consider how we feel overall as well.

0	Rest – no activity.
1	Very light activity (gentle stretching).
2	Light activity (walking slowly).
3	Light activity (walking with more pace).
4	Moderate activity (brisk walking, without being out of breath).
5	Moderate activity (brisk walking with intention).
6	Vigorous activity (jogging, increases your heart rate).
7	Vigorous activity (jogging, increases your heart rate and makes you breathe harder and faster).
8	Hard activity like running. Highest level of activity you can continue doing without stopping.
9	Very hard activity like running but can be continued for some time.
10	Maximum activity. Short bursts such as sprints or shuttle run drills that you cannot continue for long.

How hard we push ourselves during exercise depends a lot on our individual fitness level but, generally speaking, the guidelines suggest 30–45 minutes of moderate intensity exercise, 4–5 days a week.[26] This would mean exercising between numbers 4 and 6 on the RPE scale. Alternatively, as our fitness level increases we could decide to up the intensity of our exercises but reduce the length of each workout – for example, working to an exertion level of 7 or 8, but only for 20 minutes, 3 days a week.

Just before we get to the circuits and you start upping the intensity of your workouts, here's a reminder of the red flags to look out for, that might indicate you need to scale back your exercise for the time being.

1 Pain. Often we notice pain during movement if our technique is compromised. Feeling the effects of an exercise is okay, and sometimes we will notice a buildup of muscular ache during a movement, but any sharp pain or pain that doesn't subside once a movement stops is an indication that this exercise is too challenging at this time.

2 Technique. We always want to make sure we're able to maintain the correct technique for each exercise. Arching too much in the lower back, clenching your jaw or curling your toes in order to perform a movement, are all signs that an exercise is too challenging at this time.

3 Joint mobility. We know from previous chapters that our hormone levels are still up and down and that can continue for many months postpartum, longer for breastfeeding women. Being aware of how our body feels daily is important, so that we can be sure not to overload any joints still compromised by the laxity caused by pre- and postnatal hormones.

Any time you notice one of the above, simply take your exercise back a step and build up to it over time.

"WE CAN THEN BUILD UP OUR FITNESS LEVEL SLOWLY. REMEMBER, WE DON'T WANT TO RUSH RECOVERY."

Timeline recap

The American College of Obstetricians and Gynecologists (ACOG) recommends that women can begin pelvic floor exercises and low-impact walking as soon as they feel ready post-birth.[27]

Those of us who have experienced some form of assisted birth or caesarean section will be encouraged to stand and move within the first 24 hours of birth, provided that there were no further complications postpartum.

After being cleared for more exercise, usually after the 6–8 week check by the GP or midwife, we should start with optimal breathing techniques, core rehabilitation and posture realignment. We can then begin introducing the same level of exercises we were doing towards the end of our pregnancy. If you were performing press-ups with your arms on a raised platform, for example, and with your knees on the floor, then I'd recommend starting by modifying press-ups in this way again.

We can then build up our fitness level slowly. Remember, we don't want to rush recovery. If we 'skip a step' we could cause bad habits that, in the long term, might be harder for us to overcome.

Exercise circuits

On to the good stuff! The following circuits are written in progression order. All exercises are suggestions only, and always make sure you've been given the all clear to exercise by your GP or medical team first.

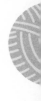

Body weight exercises: stage 1

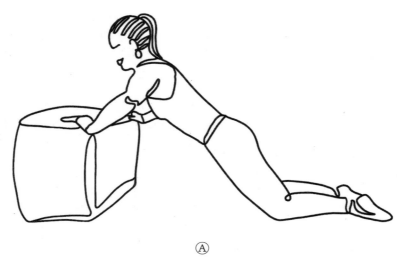

(A)

1

Elevated press-ups
Areas worked: Chest, arms and core

● Kneel in front of a secure elevated platform like a bench, garden wall or chair.

● Place both of your hands on the platform, keeping your arms extended straight out in front of you at chest height.

● Walk your knees backwards until you have reached a comfortable plank position, with optimal alignment from your neck to your tailbone. Keep your eyeline raised just in front of your hands, so that your neck stays in a straight line, avoiding dropping your chin to your chest or crunching your neck backwards.

● Inhale and bend your elbows so that your chest lowers down towards the platform (image A).

● Once your chest is a few centimetres away from the platform, exhale and push back into your plank, extending your arms so that your chest lifts back up, away from the platform.

● Inhale and repeat for 8–10 reps.

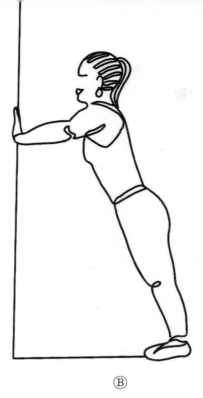

(B)

Progression and Modification

● To progress this exercise, perform the same movement in a full plank position.

● To do this, begin standing in front of the platform. Note that the higher the platform, the easier the exercise will be for your core, so you may wish to begin doing this against a wall or sideboard and progress down to a chair and eventually the floor.

● Place both of your hands on the platform, keeping your arms extended straight out in front of you at chest height (image B).

● Walk your feet backwards until you have reached a comfortable full plank position, still maintaining optimal alignment from your neck to your tailbone.

● Inhale and bend your elbows so that your chest lowers down towards the platform as in the original exercise.

● Once your chest is a few centimetres away from the platform, exhale, and pushing into your palms, straighten your arms so that your chest lifts back up, away from the platform.

● Inhale and repeat for 8–10 reps.

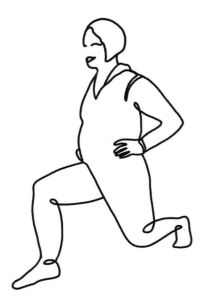

2

Forward alternate lunges
Areas worked: Legs and glutes

● Stand tall with your feet hip-width apart and your hands on your hips.

● Inhale and take a big step forwards with your left foot, immediately bending both of your knees so that both form a 90-degree angle. Your right knee should be a few centimetres off the floor with your right heel raised.

● Exhale and push off the front foot, back to the starting position.

● Inhale and repeat on the other side.

● Repeat for 8–10 reps on each side.

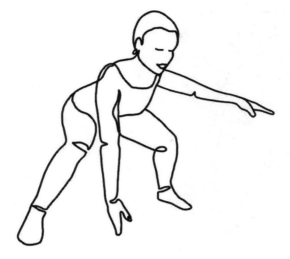

3

Side-step squat reach
Areas worked: Legs and glutes

● Stand tall with your feet hip-width apart, arms relaxed by your sides.

● Inhale and, keeping your eyeline forwards, take a step out to the side with your left foot.

● Sit backwards, bending your knees into a squat position, keeping your spine and neck neutral. Imagine you are sitting back into a chair.

● Allow your left hand to travel back naturally and your right hand to reach down to touch the floor in the middle of your two feet.

● Exhale and, with your left foot, step back into the start position.

● Inhale and immediately step out to the right with your right foot.

● As you sit back into your squat, this time allow your right arm to naturally travel back as your left hand reaches down to touch the floor in between your feet.

● Exhale and push off your right foot back to the start position.

● Continue in this way for 15–20 reps each side.

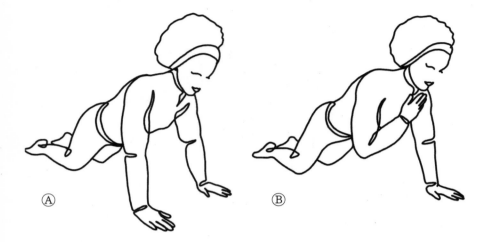

4

Modified plank with shoulder tap progression
Areas worked: Core and shoulders

● Begin on your hands and knees in the table-top position, with your hands slightly wider than shoulder-width apart and your knees directly under your hips.

● Walk your hands forwards until your body forms a straight, diagonal line from your head to your tailbone (image A).

● Keep your eyeline forwards so that your neck maintains good alignment, without tucking your chin towards your chest or crunching your neck backwards.

● Inhale and hold this position, drawing up your pelvic floor as your exhale.

● To progress this exercise, inhale and on your next exhale lift your right hand off the floor, and, crossing your chest, tap your left shoulder. Try to maintain good alignment and not let your hips tilt (image B).

● Once you have tapped your left shoulder immediately place your right hand back onto the floor and lift your left hand to cross your chest and tap your right shoulder.

● Inhale and return to the start position.

● Continue marching with your hands in this way, for 12 repetitions each side.

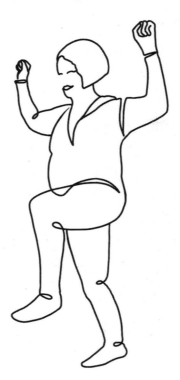

5

March with knee raise
Areas worked: Core and cardio

● Begin standing tall with your feet hip-width apart, arms relaxed by your sides.

● Inhale to prepare and bring your arms up overhead so that they are fully extended but not locked.

● As you exhale, march your knees up by first raising your right knee towards your chest, then immediately placing your right foot back down on the floor and lifting your left knee up.

● Continue alternating your knee lifts in this way.

● Simultaneously, every time you bring up a knee, draw your shoulder blades together, bringing your elbows down towards your knees. Be aware not to arch your lower back and focus on engaging your pelvic floor, maintaining a neutral spine throughout.

● Each time you inhale and lower your leg back to the floor, release your arms up overhead.

● Continue at pace for 30–40 seconds.

Body weight exercises: stage 2

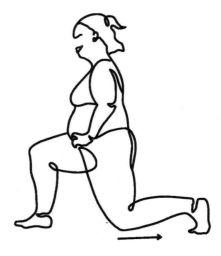

1

Reverse lunges
Areas worked: Legs and glutes

● Stand tall with your feet hip-width apart and hands on your hips.

● Inhale and take a large step backwards with your left foot to prepare.

● Lower your hips to the floor by bending both your knees to a 90-degree angle. Your right knee should be directly over your ankle and your left knee should be a few centimetres off the floor with your left heel lifted.

● Exhale and return to standing by pressing into your right heel (front foot) and pushing off your left foot bringing your left leg forwards to the start position.

● Repeat on the other side.

● Continue for 8–10 reps on each side.

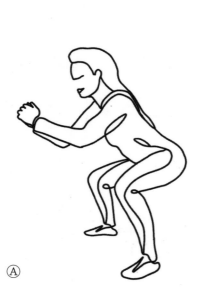

(A)

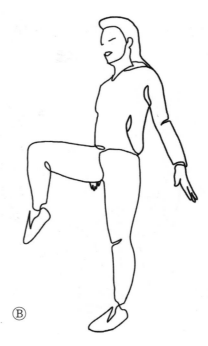

(B)

2

Squat knee raise

Areas worked: Legs, glutes and core

● Begin with your feet slightly wider than shoulder-width apart, arms relaxed by your sides.

● Inhale and sit back into a squat position.

● Simultaneously bring your hands together in front of your chest, bending your elbows (image A).

● Exhale and push up through your feet to standing.

● As you come up, immediately shift your weight onto your left leg, bringing your right knee up towards your chest, releasing your arms back to your sides (image B).

● Inhale and bring your right leg back to the floor in the start position.

● Immediately exhale and squat back down to repeat on the other side. This time, shift your weight onto your right leg as you come to standing and bring your left knee up to your chest.

● Continue alternating sides for 10–12 repetitions each side.

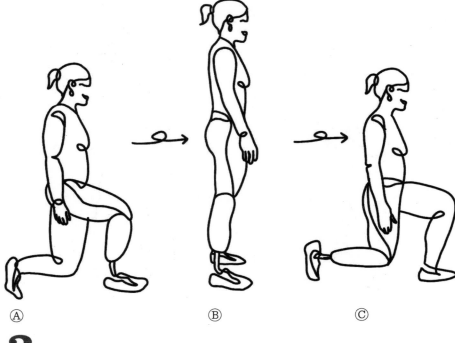

(A)   (B)   (C)

3

Kneel to standing
Areas worked: Legs, glutes and core

● Begin by kneeling on a mat with your knees stacked directly underneath your hips, your spine neutral and your arms relaxed by your sides.

● Inhale and step your right leg forwards so that the sole of your right foot is on the floor and your right knee is bent to a 90-degree angle (image A).

● Exhale and push through your right heel, bringing your left foot forwards and coming to a standing position, feet hip-width apart (image B).

● Inhale and step your right leg backwards, sinking through lunge position, immediately lowering your right knee to the floor (image C).

● Release your left foot backwards to return to the start kneeling position.

● Repeat and continue on this side for 8–10 reps before repeating with the other leg.

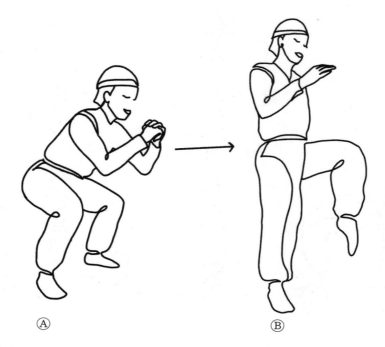

(A)   (B)

4

Squat march
Areas worked: Legs, glutes and core

● Begin standing tall, with your feet placed slightly wider than hip-width apart. Inhale and sit back into your hips as though you are going to sit down on a chair, bending your knees and sitting down as far as you can whilst keeping your chest lifted and your lower back neutral (image A).

● Exhale and push back up to the standing position.

● As you reach standing, immediately shift your weight onto your left foot, bringing your right knee towards your chest. Instantly place the right foot back on the floor and shift your weight onto your right side so that you can lift your left knee to your chest (image B).

● Place your left foot back on the ground.

● Immediately inhale and repeat the exercise.

● Continue in this way for 12–14 repetitions.

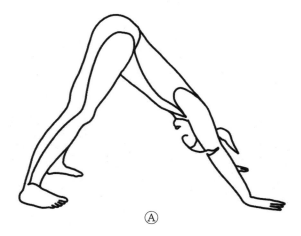

(A)

5

Downward dog to modified press-up
Areas worked: Arms, shoulders and core

Set up

● To get into the starting position for this exercise, begin by kneeling on the floor with your knees directly under your hips, arms relaxed by your sides.

● Walk your hands forwards so that you reach a half plank position, with a diagonal line running from your neck to your tailbone. Your knees should remain on the ground.

Inhale and tuck your toes under so that they are resting on the floor and push back onto your feet so that your body forms an inverted 'V'. You should now be on your hands and feet; both should be shoulder-width apart and your hips

will be raised in the air. Your heels may be slightly raised off the ground (image A).

● Your weight should be placed evenly between the front and back halves of your body.

Movement

● From this position, inhale and shift your weight forwards into your hands, pushing onto your toes and immediately lowering your knees back to the ground.

● Bend your elbows to perform a press-up, bringing your chest towards the floor, keeping your eyeline straight ahead in line with the tops of your fingertips (image B).

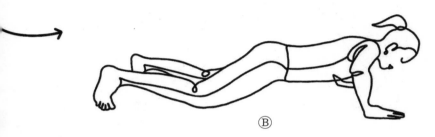

(B)

- Exhale and push through your hands, extending your arms straight. Then raise your knees off the ground and push back onto your feet to return to the inverted 'V' position.

- Repeat this movement for 8–10 repetitions before returning to the half plank position, with your knees on the ground. Walk your hands backwards until you are resting back onto your heels to recover.

Modification

To modify this exercise, you may wish to start in the inverted 'V' position with bent knees. This can help you to distribute your weight more evenly between upper and lower body if needed.

Progression

- To progress this exercise, begin in the full 'V' position as directed above.

- As you shift your weight forwards towards your hands and onto your toes, keep your knees off the floor and bend your elbows in the full press-up position. Be sure to maintain good spinal alignment, not piking your hips up or allowing them to droop down low.

- As you extend your arms, push back into the full downward dog position.

Resistance band exercises: stage 3

When I first started introducing equipment to my training, I used a resistance band. They're lightweight, portable and easy to store, and they're great for upping the intensity of a workout.

There are different types of resistance bands: cable ones, also known as tube bands; mini bands; light therapy resistance bands; figure of eight bands; and power bands, also known as loop bands. For the purpose of the below exercises we're using therapy bands. They are a long, flat elastic band that you can tie in a knot if needed.

They come in different strengths. In short, the thicker the band the more resistance it provides, and in turn the more challenging the exercise becomes.

Resistance bands usually start with level 1 and move upwards in resistance to level 6, or you might find that they're offered in a set of three – light, medium and hard. Therapy bands can vary slightly in length but they're usually around 5 feet long; however, level 1 bands will be easier to stretch so can be pulled longer, which makes them better suited to exercises that need a greater range of movement.

THE THICKER THE BAND THE MORE RESISTANCE IT PROVIDES, AND IN TURN THE MORE CHALLENGING THE EXERCISE BECOMES.

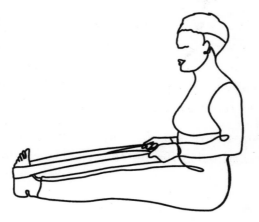

1

Resistance band row
Areas worked: Arms, back and shoulders

BAND STRENGTH: LIGHT–MEDIUM

● Begin in a seated position on the floor, with your legs straight out in front of you.

● Holding on to each end of the resistance band, with your palms facing each other, place the centre of the band around your feet.

● Inhale to prepare and sit tall.

● As you exhale, engage your pelvic floor and draw your elbows directly back so that they brush past your sides, until your fists reach your sides and your elbows are behind you.

● Inhale and slowly release your arms forwards into an extended position. Avoid rounding your back and maintain optimal posture throughout.

● Repeat for 12–16 repetitions.

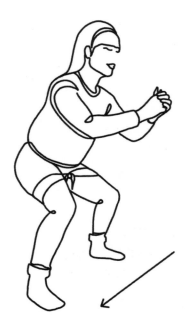

2

Travelling squats
Areas worked: Legs and glutes

BAND STRENGTH: LIGHT–MEDIUM

Using a resistance band for this exercise will help us focus more on the eccentric part of the movement, which means working a muscle as it is lengthened. Research shows that this way of training can have great benefits. We just need to be aware of our breathing and concentrate on performing a slow, controlled movement, using our breath to draw up our pelvic floor on the down phase.

You will need enough space to move sideways about 10–20 paces for this exercise.

● Tie your resistance band in a knot and step into the loop, pulling the band up to your thighs. Flatten out the band around your legs and keep the knot in the middle of your thighs at the front.

● Prepare for the exercise by standing up with your feet slightly wider than hip-width apart. You may wish to turn your feet out a fraction, about 15 degrees.

● You should feel a light resistance from the band already in this position. If needed, readjust the knot in the band to get the right length for this.

● When you're ready, inhale to prepare.

● As you exhale, take a step out with your left leg to your left side.

● Draw up your pelvic floor as you sit back into your hips as though you are sitting onto an invisible chair. Bend your knees and sit back as far as you can or until your thighs are parallel with the floor, whilst keeping your spine neutral and your chest up. You should feel the resistance working against your legs; continue to push into that sensation.

● Inhale and push through both of your heels, bringing your right foot back in to standing with your feet hip-width apart.

● Exhale and repeat the movement, moving continually to your left.

● Focus on drawing up the pelvic floor as you lower into your squat, thereby working the muscle eccentrically.

● Repeat for 8 repetitions to your left and then perform the same 8 on the other side.

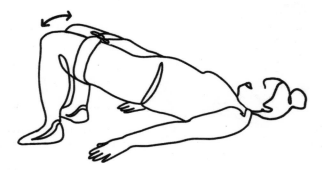

3

Glute bridge pulses
Areas worked: Glutes and lower back

BAND STRENGTH: MEDIUM

● Sit on a mat, tie your resistance band in a knot and pull the band up to your thighs.

● Lie back onto the mat, with your knees bent so that the soles of your feet are flat on the floor, hip-width apart. Your arms should be relaxed by your sides and the resistance band should be flat around your thighs with the knot in the middle of your legs at the front.

● You should feel a light resistance from the band already in this position. If needed, readjust the knot in the band to get the right length for this.

● Inhale to prepare, and as you exhale draw up your pelvic floor and engage your glutes so that your hips are lifted off the floor.

● Raise your hips and work against the resistance you feel from the band until your hips are straight and you have created a diagonal line from your tailbone down to your shoulders on the floor.

● In this position breathe freely and pulse slightly outwards with both knees, by engaging your glutes and increasing the resistance through the band. Repeat for 10–12 pulses. Then inhale and release your hips back down to the start position on the floor.

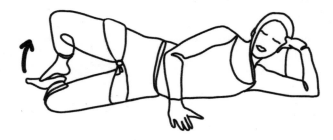

4

Clam
Areas worked: Glutes

BAND STRENGTH: MEDIUM

● Tie your resistance band in a knot and pull the band up to your thighs.

● Lie on your left side with your legs stacked and knees bent to a 45-degree angle.

● Rest your left arm along the floor, then bend your left elbow and lift your forearm up so that you can support your head with your hand. Use your right arm to steady your frame by placing your hand on your right hip or gently resting it on the floor in front of you. Be aware of keeping on your side and not rolling forwards.

● Your resistance band should be flattened out around your thighs with the knot between your legs at the front.

● Inhale to prepare, and as you exhale draw up your pelvic floor.

● As you engage your glutes, lift your top knee towards the ceiling, keeping your feet together and keeping your lower leg on the ground.

● Hold this clam position with your legs for 2–3 seconds.

● Inhale and release the top knee back to the start position.

● Repeat for 10–12 repetitions.

5

Tricep extension
Areas worked: Triceps

BAND STRENGTH: LIGHT

Set up

● Begin standing in a small split-legged stance. Looking forwards, your left foot should be about one foot in front of your right, but maintaining a hip-width distance between them.

● Stand on one end of your resistance band with your back (right) foot. Keep hold of the other end with your right hand.

● As you stand, the band should be partially stretched behind you. Bring your right arm up so that your elbow is bent to the side of your head, with your fist behind you, in line with your shoulder.

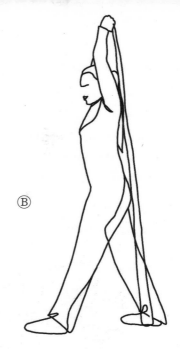

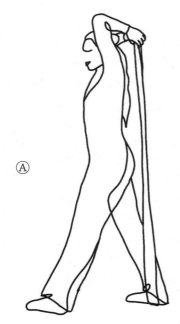

● Bring your left hand to join your right, holding on to the resistance band (image A).

● Be aware that your head and neck are in a neutral position and not shifting forwards, straining your neck.

Movement

● Holding the resistance band in your fists, inhale to prepare, and as you exhale extend your arms straight up overhead. This should stretch the resistance band further and you should feel the tension in your arms (image B).

● Inhale and release tension in the band by bending your elbows and lowering your hands back down towards your shoulders.

● Repeat for 10–12 repetitions.

● If you wish to perform another set, you can swap your feet around, bringing your right foot in front and your left foot back as the anchor for the band.

Dumbbell workout: stage 4

Dumbbell workouts can seem intimidating if you haven't used weights before, but they're such a great way to progress our exercises and can actually be a lot of fun. Hopefully you enjoy it and you'll soon see the benefits in your strength, toning and fitness level, as well as better coordination and stability of muscles and joints.

Here's a great dumbbell circuit for beginners, with progressions for anyone who is more experienced. How heavy you should lift will depend on your fitness level, but I would generally recommend choosing a set of weights between 3 and 7kg. If you have multiple weights, opt for one lighter set and one heavier set to give yourself variation.

'DUMBBELL WORKOUTS CAN SEEM INTIMIDATING IF YOU HAVEN'T USED WEIGHTS BEFORE, BUT THEY'RE SUCH A GREAT WAY TO PROGRESS OUR EXERCISES AND CAN ACTUALLY BE A LOT OF FUN.'

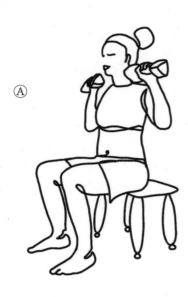

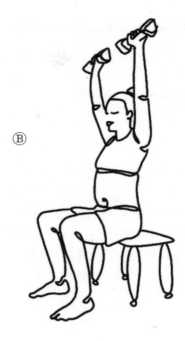

1

Seated shoulder press
Areas worked: Shoulders and back

● Sit on a bench or chair, holding onto a dumbbell in each hand, using a neutral grip (palms facing inwards), with your arms relaxed by your sides.

● Sit with a neutral posture so that you allow the three curves of your spine to sit naturally.

● To prepare, bend your elbows and rotate the dumbbells so that your palms are now in front of your shoulders, with your fists facing the front. Your dumbbells should now be horizontal facing outwards (image A).

● Inhale to prepare, and as you exhale and draw up your pelvic floor, push the dumbbells straight up overhead so that your arms are fully extended but not locked. Be careful not to crunch your shoulders and neck and instead focus on keeping your shoulders back and down (image B).

● Inhale and bend your elbows so that the dumbbells return to shoulder height.

● Exhale and push the dumbbells back overhead.

● Repeat for 8–10 repetitions.

Progression: Squat shoulder press

(Note: in this progression the exhale occurs as you push to standing.)

● To progress this exercise prepare in a similar way to the seated shoulder press above.

● Sit comfortably on a chair, keeping good postural alignment. Bend your elbows so that your fists are resting just in front of your shoulders, but this time keep your fists facing in towards one another (image A).

● Inhale and, as you exhale, draw up your pelvic floor and engage your glutes as you push up to a standing position. Simultaneously press your dumbbells overhead so that your arms are straight but not locked (image B).

● Inhale and bring your arms back down so that your dumbbells are resting just in front of your shoulders. Sit back into your squat until you are resting back in the start position, seated on the chair. Continue in this way and repeat for 8–10 repetitions.

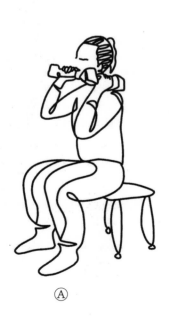

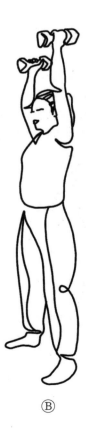

Ⓐ   Ⓑ

2

Travelling lunges
Areas worked: Legs and glutes

● Begin by standing tall, holding on to your dumbbells with a neutral grip with your palms facing inwards. Your feet should be hip-width apart.

● Bend your elbows and bring the dumbbells up so that they are positioned in front of your shoulders, this time with your palms facing inwards towards each other.

● Take a wide step forwards with your left foot, sinking into a lunge so that your knees are bent to a 90-degree angle with your front knee over your ankle and your back knee a few centimetres off the floor with your right heel raised (image A).

● Return to standing by pushing through your front heel and bringing your back leg forwards to meet your front leg, maintaining a hip-width distance.

● Repeat by stepping forwards with the other leg.

● Continue alternating and moving forwards for 8 reps each side.

Progression: with shoulder press

● To progress this exercise, begin in the same standing position as above.

● Step forwards and as you bend down into your lunge, push your dumbbells overhead so that your arms are fully extended but not locked (image B).

● Inhale, and as you come to a standing position bring your dumbbells back down to shoulder height.

● Continue to press your dumbbells overhead in this way for the duration of the exercise.

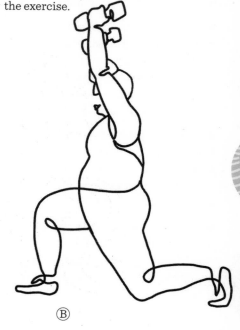

Ⓐ   Ⓑ

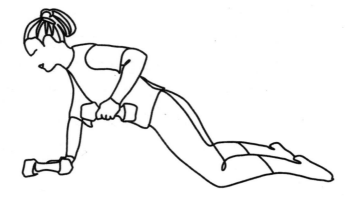

3

Modified plank row
Areas worked: Back, shoulders, triceps, biceps and core

● Begin in the modified plank position with your dumbbells lying parallel on the floor between your hands. Your knees should be bent and your arms should be fully extended just in front of your chest, shoulder-width apart.

● Shift your weight forwards so that you are in the half plank position, forming a straight diagonal line from your neck to your tailbone, maintaining a neutral spine position.

● Inhale to prepare, and grasp the left dumbbell in your left hand. As you exhale, draw up your pelvic floor and simultaneously lift your left elbow back

until your hand is level with your ribs. Keep your arm close to your ribcage so that you brush past your side.

● Keep your plank still and your hips stable.

● Inhale and extend your left arm back to the start position.

● On your next exhale repeat the movement with the same arm, drawing your elbow back and keeping it close to your chest.

● Inhale as you return to the start position.

YOU'LL SOON SEE THE BENEFITS, INCLUDING MUSCLE GROWTH, STRENGTH AND TONING, AS WELL AS BETTER COORDINATION AND STABILITY OF MUSCLES AND JOINTS.

● Repeat this rowing movement for 10–12 repetitions, without losing the stability of your plank.

● Repeat on the other side.

Progression: full plank

(Note: this is an intermediate to advanced-level exercise)

● To progress this exercise, perform your rows from a full plank position.

● In order to achieve this, begin with your arms slightly wider than shoulder-width apart, walk your feet back until your legs are fully extended and you are grounded through your toes on both feet. You may prefer to have your feet wider than hip-width apart to help with stability.

● Maintain a neutral spine and stabilise your hips throughout the rowing motion.

● With each exhale, draw up your pelvic floor as you row your elbow back.

● Continue to row for 8 repetitions before resting and then repeating on the other side.

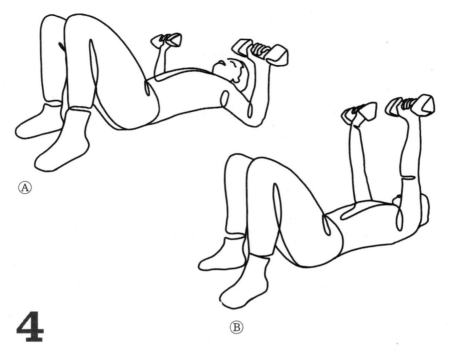

(A)

(B)

4

Chest press
Areas worked: Chest, biceps and triceps

● Lie back on the floor with your knees bent so that the soles of your feet are flat on the floor, hip-width apart.

● Hold your dumbbells with a neutral grip and bend your elbows so that your forearms come off the floor. Your dumbbells should now be raised off the ground with your fists facing each other in line with your chest.

● Rotate your arms slightly so that your fists are facing outwards and your dumbbells are horizontal (image A).

● Inhale to prepare, and as you exhale draw up your pelvic floor and push your dumbbells straight up in front of you, straightening your arms but not locking them (image B).

● Inhale and slowly lower your elbows back down.

● Just as your elbows brush the ground, exhale and repeat the press up in front of you.

● Continue this motion for 12–20 repetitions.

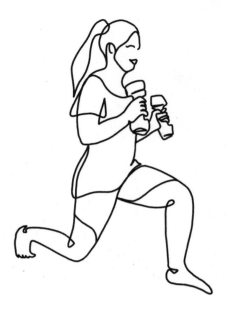

5

Reverse lunge with dumbbell curl
Areas worked: Legs, glutes, core, biceps and triceps

● Begin standing tall with your feet hip-width apart, holding the dumbbells at your sides with a neutral grip.

● Inhale to prepare, and as you exhale take a wide step backwards with your right foot and bend both of your knees to a 90-degree angle. Simultaneously bend both of your elbows so that your dumbbells curl up towards your shoulders.

● Make sure that your left knee (front) is directly over your ankle. The heel of your right foot will be off the floor.

● Inhale and push through the heel of your left (front) foot and come to standing, returning to the start position. As you do this, uncurl your arms and lower your dumbbells back down to your sides.

● Repeat this movement on the other side by stepping back with your left foot. As you lower back, your right foot (now at the front) should be over your knee and your left heel will be off the floor.

● Continue to curl both elbows up with each lunge.

● Alternate sides and repeat for 10 reps each side.

Cueing yourself

Getting your cues right for exercises is probably one of the more challenging aspects of self-training. Saying the wrong cue to ourselves over and over can trigger an incorrect visualisation, which might trickle down into how an exercise is performed.

For example, simply thinking 'suck in your abs' won't create the same effect as thinking 'draw up your pelvic floor'. Both have the same goal; however, the second will allow a more well-rounded activation leading to much more effective results.

Here are a few more important body cues to consider.

Posture

Ever been told to 'stand tall' in the past, or 'not to slouch'? Well, instead of simply thinking 'stand tall', which could lead to a tense, rigid feeling, we'd be much better served by visualising ourselves being 'suspended' from the ceiling. This way we will hopefully achieve a 'lightness' to our posture. By visualising our head being drawn up by a string in the air, we get a sense that we should be upright but can still move, mobile and free, keeping our chest elevated and body light.

Shoulders

Ever heard someone say, 'Engage your shoulders back and down'? Well, this is great during an exercise, but we can't spend all day focusing on engaging our back muscles. What we can do, however, is be aware of not crunching up our shoulders towards our neck. A good cue would be 'release your shoulders'. This way we are encouraged to release any tension we might be carrying in our upper back. Take a deep inhale and do a few shoulder rolls backwards. Tilt your head side to side. Perhaps place one hand on your opposite shoulder, push your shoulder up into your hand for a few seconds and then release. Notice how much tension flows out of your neck and shoulder as a result.

Butt-gripping

I can hardly write this with a straight face, but I'm seeing a crisis occurring in the postnatal world of butt-gripping. This refers to 'clenching' of the buttocks. Take a moment now to think, can you release your glutes? Are you clenching without even realising it? I would wager that you are. In general, most people could do with glute release work.

During exercises it's common to hear instructors tell their clients to 'squeeze' their glutes, but in fact we should be encouraging our ladies to 'draw in' their glutes and always make sure we emphasise the need to release again afterwards.

Knees

Look down from your pelvis and you'll find knees and feet. Needless to say, it's all linked. By that reasoning it makes sense that we should all check in with our leg alignment once in a while. The cue 'stand straight' can instantly make people lock their knees. Locking your knees in exercise puts maximum pressure and stress on the knee joint. Similarly, sitting with your knees at a 90-degree angle for long periods of time can irritate the joint. Knees need to move. This is why standing up and changing our position regularly is recommended, as well as keeping in mind the suspended sensation we discussed for optimum posture.

Hopefully this chapter has shed some light on how to safely progress exercises in the postpartum period. Listening to your body and trusting your instincts are key; however, if you have any concerns be sure to raise them with your medical team or reach out to a specialist trainer and ask for advice. Coming up, we look at how best to get back into running after birth, and how it was written into human nature millions of years ago. Don't be put off if you don't consider yourself a running enthusiast. You might just find that a spark of interest is ignited within the coming pages.

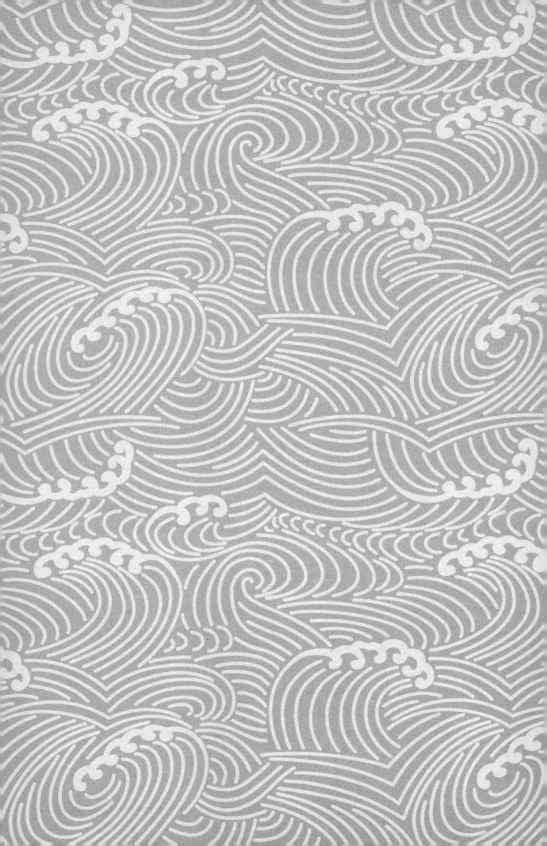

Returning to running postpartum

Humans were born to run.

It's been part of our instinctive human nature for more than two million years – at least that's what the experts believe after looking back at fossil evidence.

History and science show us that after standing up, humans eventually evolved into endurance runners. In fact, some scientists are even adamant that this is the very reason the human body looks as it does today.

I gave running its own chapter because it's meant so much to me since motherhood. Although I've always enjoyed it, it wasn't until motherhood that I found just how healing the motion can be. It became less painful and much more fun and relaxing.

I know that for some people even the word 'running' makes them nervous. If you don't run 5km minimum you're not a runner, right? Wrong! Let me assure you, if you put on a pair of trainers and head out the door, you're officially a runner. No matter if you're stop-starting, or if you're mostly walking, you are still a runner. Whether you run 2 minutes, 2 miles or 2 hours, it all counts and you're still a runner!

Born to run

'Running is one of the transformational events in human history,' according to Dennis Bramble, a biology professor at the University of Utah who has studied human evolution in detail.[28] So much so, in fact, that it's argued that 'the emergence of humans is tied to the evolution of running' – which means our ability to run played a pivotal part in the expansion and sustainability of the entire human race.

Running kept our ancestors alive and cemented our place in the food chain. It was one of the ways that Mother Nature began to distinguish us homo sapiens from our tree-dwelling predecessors, allowing us to leave them behind and hunt further afield.

The development of our ancestors into long-distance runners helped them to compete with much speedier carnivores on the plains of Africa and hunt down prey. They weren't as fast as cheetahs, but they could outlast them.

Although this might sound like ancient history, there are still tribes present on Earth today that have retained the ability to hunt prey in this way. The San Bushmen from southern Africa can outrun horses or antelopes over extremely long distances. As Bramble says, 'Even more important than pure speed is combining reasonable speed with exceptional endurance.'

Granted, when I hobble around my 5km, I certainly don't feel so invincible or have much endurance left at the end, but we can't argue with the fact that running and movement is in our DNA. It's a skill we were born with; we just need to rediscover it and set our animal instinct free.

I do understand that it may feel impossible to fit running into your busy schedule. Let's face it, in many countries today, running is regarded as a leisure activity, not something our body needs to survive.

But movement isn't just a leisure activity; it's a necessity. Our body and our brain need it! So why, when it's so important to our health to move or run, do we at times still feel apprehensive about giving running a go?

Running for modern-day mamas

Aside from labour, running is probably one of the few times when I have felt my most primal. I think that's part of what connects me to the sport. I get a reminder of what motherhood is like. At times it's tough, but it's also exhilarating and always worth it. And sometimes it's just the best medicine for my body and brain.

From listening to friends and clients over the years, I think what puts many people off is that running can sometimes feel hard. I suppose there's no escaping that it can certainly be challenging when you push yourself, but that's true of anything if we want to improve, right? I think running in particular can feel testing because no matter how much we improve, we're likely to always stretch our limits.

For example, if you usually jog at about 60 or 70 per cent of your maximum effort, no matter how fit you become, if you keep pushing yourself to 70 per cent, the intensity of the exercise will feel consistently challenging. It might feel like you're not improving when in actual fact you are.

As for running after pregnancy and birth, I have returned to running three times now and every time I've enjoyed it more.

If I'm honest, running gives me a break from the chaos, allows my brain to relax and my body to breathe. It has nothing to do with how fast or far I've run. I've had days where I've run a 10km in under an hour or taken over an hour to run 5km. I've walked, hobbled, sprinted, jogged and stopped. All of those times, I enjoyed running!

Running doesn't need to be about hitting targets. We can find the fun, if we relax into the motion and absorb the benefits.

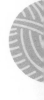

So, what exactly are the benefits of running for mums?

I'll stick to giving you the facts. Hopefully they might tip the scale for anyone who's on the brink of giving running a go.

Running is a wonder workout. It's the avocado of exercise. A super-mover if you will. The benefits transcend body and mind, and the physical effects reach our muscles, joints and posture!

Jogging is a form of aerobic exercise, which literally means 'with oxygen'. It uses our cardiovascular system, increasing our heart rate, which keeps our heart, lungs and circulatory system healthy. Most people know it simply as 'cardio'.

It's a great fat-burning exercise too, helping to lower cholesterol levels and assist with muscle tone. As a weight-bearing exercise, running also helps improve our bone health, reset hormone levels and improve neurological function within the brain. This simple exercise increases our overall health and is even shown to extend our lifespan.

As a mum, I found running also had a new benefit I hadn't fully appreciated before: it gave me time to myself. I have jogged with a stroller, but I'll admit, I enjoy it more alone. For me, running is a moment where I can fully immerse myself in being me. It's not often for long but any running is better than no running.

The endurance aspect

Speaking as someone who has always preferred short sprints to endurance running, I struggled to get to grips with longer distances.

My husband is one of those people who has always been able to jump out of bed any random morning and, at the drop of a hat, run 10km. He needs little to no preparation and just seems able to run with ease. I, on the other hand, have to work at it.

The reason for this comes down to the make-up of our muscle fibres. Everyone has both long- and short-twitch muscle fibres. Long (slow) twitch muscle fibres are better suited to support endurance movements, like marathons, whereas short (fast)-twitch fibres assist shorter and faster movements, like sprints. Our muscles contain both fast- and slow-twitch fibres, but the ratio of how many of each type we have can change and we can train ourselves to develop more of each type too.

It's amazing how quickly our body can adapt and improve in a short space of time. When I returned to running after my twin pregnancy, I only managed an average of one, maximum two runs a week, yet I still noticed improvements within weeks.

Which are you?

Your muscle fibres won't just be slow- or fast-twitch as everyone has a combination of both, but the ratio of muscle fibres you have will depend on factors like your genetics, age and style of training. To a degree, we can train ourselves to shift the ratio in the direction we want.

People leading sedentary lifestyles (with minimal movement) are said to have roughly a 50–50 split of muscle fibres. Professional sprint athletes have roughly 75 per cent fast-twitch fibres, whereas marathon runners have between 70 and 80 per cent slow-twitch.

Without delving too deep, it's worth noting that slow-twitch muscle fibres use a combination of oxygen, fat and a stored form of energy in our bodies called glycogen to function, but our fast-twitch fibres run off our anaerobic energy system. You might know of it as your lactic acid system. This gets its name from the fact that when we use different forms of energy stored in our muscles, without the presence of oxygen, we produce lactic acid in our muscles.

This system is basically a process our body uses to make energy quickly. It gives us powerful energy fast, but it burns up quickly as well, which is why our fast-twitch muscle fibres fatigue much quicker. This is also why a sprint will have us lying flat out within a minute or less, but long-distance runners can continue for miles.

Important muscles like our heart and those in our legs, back and core consist more of slow-twitch fibres because they need to keep us moving and upright all day every day.

Age can also be a factor. As we age, the amount of lean muscle mass we have decreases, causing a decline in our muscle fibre development. Resistance training can combat this decline to a certain extent.

If you want to increase your slow-twitch (endurance) muscle fibres, they can be developed through exercises that involve low resistance, low intensity, high repetition and long duration. This is also true if you're lifting weights. In short, if you want more endurance muscle fibres, lift lighter for longer!

If you want to pick up speed or improve your fast-twitch muscle fibres, you'll want to focus on generating force quickly. Jumping, sprinting and shorter reps of higher weights in strength training can all help with this.

How to start running after giving birth

Okay, so the passionate prologue is over, now on to the step-by-step guide on how to actually begin running after giving birth – because, let's keep it real, that first post-birth run is unlike any other running challenge!

When it comes to running during pregnancy, the current recommendations say that if you're already a runner you can continue throughout the trimesters, provided there are no medical complications. Personally, I would always still recommend keeping the intensity down to 60–70 per cent of your maximum daily effort, no matter what trimester, and in the run-up to labour you might want to reduce this even further.

I managed to run consistently throughout my first two pregnancies; however, with my twins I tried once, at around 20 weeks, and it just didn't feel right, so I knew I needed to pause any running until after delivery. As always, listening to how our body feels is the most important thing. We need to be confident in making a decision that is right for us.

In the weeks leading up to labour we should also be aware of the increased pressure already placed on our pelvic floor and front abdominal wall. Running takes good core control, so we should be mindful not to increase that pressure with too much impact exercise. This isn't to say running is out of the question, but staying aware of our supporting muscle groups allows us to manage intra-abdominal pressure. We should stop if we feel our deep core might be overstressed by the motion.

Regardless of whether you've run regularly during pregnancy or never lace up, working up to your first postpartum run isn't just a hop, skip and a jump; there are a few things we need in place first.

1 Core control

Once we've rehabilitated our deep core muscles (Chapter 10), we need to start practising putting our core under pressure during movement. Running is effectively a single-leg exercise and that takes huge amounts of core control, so it's not purely strength but also core stability we need to focus on. The following two exercises are great to begin challenging your core in different ways and encourage engagement of the deep core.

Single-leg lateral hold

● Stand tall with your feet hip-width apart, arms relaxed by your sides.

● Take a small step out to the side with your right leg and bend your right knee a little.

● Simultaneously bring your left arm forwards so that your left hand is in line with your right knee (image A).

● Inhale to prepare and as you exhale, push back laterally onto your left leg, bringing your left arm up overhead.

● You should now be standing on one leg, with your right leg bent underneath you (image B).

● Hold this position for 10 seconds if possible before returning to the start position.

● Repeat on the other side.

● Try five sets on each side.

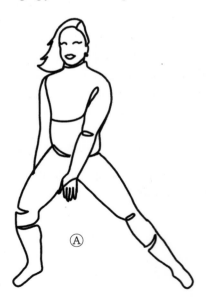

Ⓐ

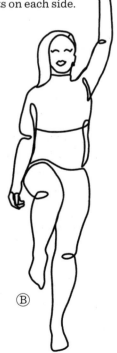

Ⓑ

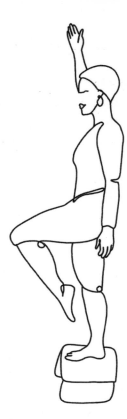

Step up hold exercise

● Stand in front of a low platform such as a step bench or garden step, no higher than 20cm. Make sure that the platform is wide enough for the full length of your foot to be supported.

● Begin stepping up onto the platform by using your left leg first, followed immediately by your right. Step down again with your left leg first, followed by your right.

● Continue stepping up and down in this way.

● Once you have achieved a steady rhythm, after about ten to fifteen steps, take a sudden stop after placing the left foot onto the platform, holding a single leg position. Hold the right foot off the step temporarily.

● Hold this position for 8–10 seconds if possible, drawing up your pelvic floor and engaging your glutes and surrounding deep core muscles to support the hold.

● Step back down to the floor and repeat the exercise on the other side.

● Continue switching sides for 6–8 reps each side.

2 Mama knows breast

Buy a good sports bra. I mentioned in Chapter 12 that breast-bouncing ranges between 3 and 5cm and that investing in a high-support bra could cut this range in half.

We might not be able to eliminate breast bouncing completely, but the goal is to assist your breasts in moving in synergy with your torso, helping to create a rhythm when running.

If you're thinking of throwing on your old bra, or maybe doubling up for extra support, I can say firsthand that it just doesn't work. Doubling up can restrict our breathing capacity, and an old bra won't be set to accommodate our new shape after the changes of pregnancy.

There are lots of options for nursing bras, which offer high support, but I've always found that while they're good for workouts, it can be tricky to find a bra that offers enough support for a run.

Breastfeeding mothers might choose to express before running, which I always found made things a little more comfortable and also left a supply of milk at home, in case one of the babies wanted feeding whilst I was away. That also meant I didn't need to choose from the somewhat limited selection of nursing bras and could instead purchase a larger-sized, high-support bra which offered good support and helped to avoid chafing.

3 Route

This one didn't occur to me initially, but I learned from experience (and embarrassment) how important route choice is for postnatal running. They say that with parenting you learn on the job, and getting stuck in the middle of the woods with a grumpy toddler provided some lessons that I will never forget!

Lesson one: if you're running with a stroller choose flat and even surfaces.

Lesson two: always make sure you know where the nearest toilet is.

Initially, we want to stick with straightforward routes and wait until we've had a chance to build strength in our deep core, legs and core support muscles before increasing the intensity of our runs. Hill running, trekking and racing at high speeds all take training, which we can work up to over the course of a few months or the first year postpartum.

4 Feet facts

Your feet are always talking to you. Are you listening?

Our feet are the first point of contact with the ground when we walk or run, so it makes sense that our foot health is important if we want to improve.

Running is essentially a single-leg exercise; both feet never hit the floor at the same time, and single-leg work takes a huge amount of pelvic and core stability. We know already from Chapter 3 that our feet are linked to our core via the deep front line (page 29) and how our feet hit the floor changes the way our body absorbs the impact of running, changing how that shock passes through the rest of our body.

During pregnancy our natural foot arches may become flattened, because of the increased weight our growing baby and uterus continually push onto our feet as we stand. I hadn't experienced this until my twin pregnancy, which is common because the pressure on our feet is greater in twin or multiple pregnancies than a singleton.

Having flat feet changes the dynamic of each step we take. My first run attempt post-twin pregnancy made me feel alien in my own skin. I couldn't understand why each step felt laboured. I couldn't lift my leg back off the ground without huge amounts of effort. I felt like I was plodding, and it felt hard and slow. I realise now that it was because of the way my feet were hitting the ground. Landing with a flat foot offers no push back off the ground, which makes running feel a lot harder. Every step is like starting from zero, as opposed to building up a rhythm.

These exercises can help us to re-establish the arch in our foot. You should notice a difference within a few months.

Finally, it might help to temporarily go up a shoe size. As the arch of your foot flattens, the soles of your feet can expand and getting the right size shoe offers much better support whilst we rehab our fallen arches.

❛DURING PREGNANCY OUR NATURAL FOOT ARCHES MAY BECOME FLATTENED, BECAUSE OF THE INCREASED WEIGHT OUR GROWING BABY AND UTERUS CONTINUALLY PUSH ONTO OUR FEET AS WE STAND.❜

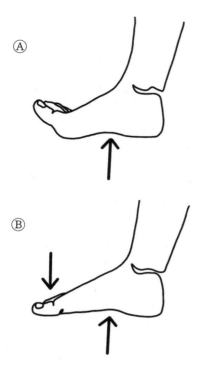

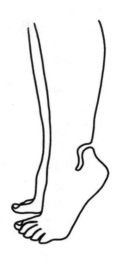

Toe lifts

● Stand tall with your feet hip-width apart, holding onto a sideboard for support if needed.

● Inhale and lift all your toes off the ground on your right foot; this will instantly create a small lift in the arch of your foot (image A).

● Hold this position for a slow count of six.

● On the next exhale, slowly lower your toes back to the ground, whilst focusing on maintaining the arch in your foot (image B).

● Inhale and release the foot, letting the entire foot relax.

Calf raises

● Stand tall with your feet hip-width apart, holding on to a sideboard for support if needed.

● Inhale, and as you exhale, lift your heels off the floor so that you rise up onto your toes.

● Inhale at the top of the movement and as you exhale, slowly lower back down until the soles of your feet are flat to the floor.

5 Posture and running

Our posture also affects our foot placement. Nursing positions can create 'bad habits' with our posture so we want to be mindful of how we're sitting and standing. It's also not uncommon for the increased size of our breasts to shift our shoulders into a rounded position, hunching our upper back, which can pull our body weight forwards.

Alongside all the exercises in Chapter 10, the below shoulder release and upper back strengthening exercises can help to encourage optimal posture and a happy alignment.

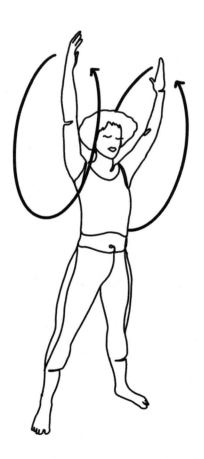

Shoulder release exercise

● Stand tall with your feet shoulder-width apart, arms relaxed by your sides.

● Inhale and swing both your arms forwards and then up overhead.

● Exhale and immediately allow them to release backwards, completing a full circle as they rest back down at your sides.

● Continue this circular motion with deep breaths for a few minutes and feel any tension in your shoulders release.

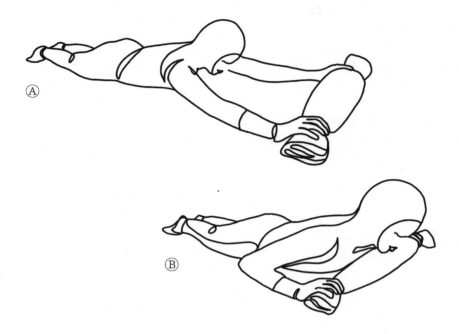

Flat row

This is an upper back exercise, specifically targeting our trapezius and latissimus dorsi muscles. You will need a rolled-up towel.

● Lie on your front on a mat, with your arms extended out in front of you.

● Hold onto your rolled-up towel with both hands, keeping your arms just wider than shoulder-width apart (image A).

● Keep your gaze just in front of you, so that you maintain good alignment from your neck to your tailbone.

● Inhale and, as you exhale, draw your elbows backwards, bending your arms so that your shoulder blades are drawn together. At the same time, draw up your pelvic floor.

● Both hands and the towel should move towards you until the towel rests just underneath your chin. Lift your chest up off the floor slightly (image B).

● Hold this position for 2–3 seconds.

● Inhale and release your arms forwards to the start position.

● Repeat for 8–10 reps.

6 Hydration

We should always sustain good hydration levels but this is particularly important for pregnant or breastfeeding women. Our body needs water to keep all the functions it's working on ticking over. Not to mention maintaining supplies of amniotic fluid or breastmilk.

Running and sweating can deplete our reserves if we don't regularly top them up. Avoid gulping one big drink immediately after a run and instead try small sips during a workout or make sure you've hydrated before setting out for a jog.

Remember, the average daily fluid intake is 8–10 glasses of water a day for prenatal women (page 211) and anywhere from 750ml to 2 litres for breastfeeding women (page 190). We want to make sure we consume this as a minimum and drink additional water any time we exercise.

7 Posture and prams

From personal experience I know that running with a buggy and a baby can take some getting used to.

I was an experienced runner and didn't think I'd have any trouble. I was excited to get out with my brand-new running pram ... but wow, my first attempt was catastrophic!

Halfway round, the front wheel just clean fell off. Turns out I hadn't attached it properly. After a lot of swearing I called my husband who brought an allen key to bolt it back on properly. I should have known then that, although I was an experienced runner, I was a total novice at buggy-running. But I started up again, determined to finish the second half strong. Unfortunately, I found that I fumbled around every corner. Now that pesky front wheel wouldn't turn at all! I stopped and examined it, hoping that my baby would hold on to his patience for a few more minutes, but no matter what I did, it wasn't turning for love nor money. So, I tried a few more minutes of jogging in as straight a line as possible, which is tricky when you live off a roundabout. I had to stop each time I encountered a corner to lift and rotate the front end of the buggy around each bend. Eventually I gave up and walked, which, incidentally, was also very tricky with this jogging stroller.

I found out later on that a locked front wheel is actually designed specifically for running strollers. The locking feature creates a cushioning effect for your baby over bumpy terrain. But it means that we need to steer the pram completely differently to how we'd direct a normal buggy.

When the front wheel is locked, we need to use our whole body weight to lean into a corner as we approach it, steering the pram by encouraging pressure down one side, so that it gently glides around the corner. This type of weight-shift steering is better done at running pace and won't work as smoothly when we're walking. This is why lots of prams have a double feature, giving you the option of a locked or swivelling front wheel.

If you want to run with a stroller, the steering is actually incredibly easy once you get the hang of it. However, you'll also want to choose a system with an adjustable handle height or a height that supports optimum posture. We know that our posture is pulled off centre during pregnancy and postnatally we want to do everything we can to get things back on track.

Let me round up this chapter by saying that I really hope that, if you do give running a go, you find the enjoyment in it. Running for me is a great mental release. It's something I like to do on my own and it gives me some much-needed time away from the pressures of parenting.

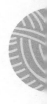

It doesn't have to take a long time and it doesn't cost the Earth. We can all throw on a pair of trainers and step out for a quick 10–20 minutes. Honestly, that's all it takes!

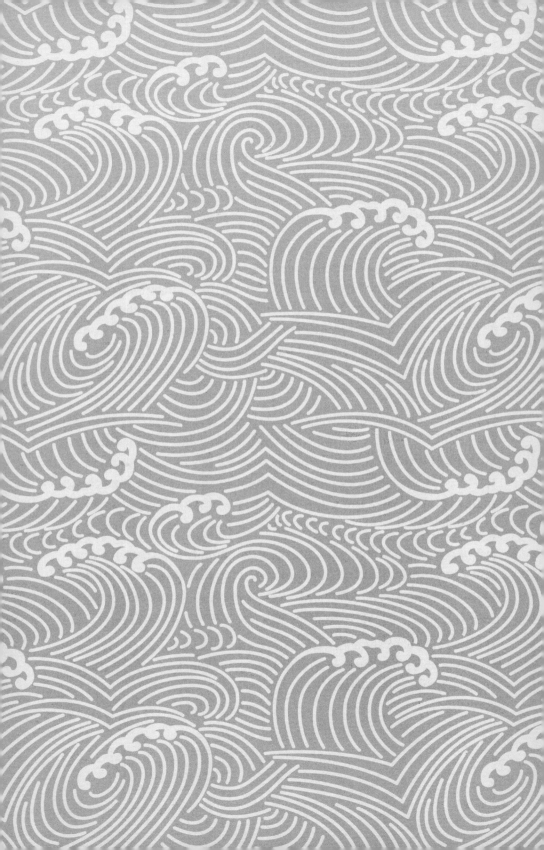

Confidence

I think the most confident I've ever felt in my life was after becoming a mum. It was almost as though I let go of all my insecurities because I didn't want my children to be held back in the same way. If I was going to encourage them to be exactly who they are and to be proud of that, I needed to live that truth myself first.

That's not to say that I've never suffered any setbacks; there have been plenty of times when I felt out of my depth. Along with the highs, motherhood has presented a ton of moments where I felt truly overwhelmed, but I always picked myself up and carried on, somehow with more confidence from having shown myself that I could in fact persevere and do it.

But self-belief is different for all of us. In writing this chapter I'm aware that my personal journey is only one experience out of countless others.

Personally, I think it's long overdue that we respect the authority of each individual woman following her birth. Even though we might feel that we share similarities with someone else's birth story, we will all experience the impact of these moments differently. We should give one another the space to be heard and, equally, we should be able to speak out for ourselves too.

Inner contentment and calm

I remember watching a Red Table talk one evening whilst breastfeeding my twins. In this episode Will Smith and Jada Pinkett Smith talked about a time in their lives when both of them felt unhappy. They did what many of us would do and turned to their closest family and friends, trying to seek support and encouragement to help them feel better. In an interesting twist, they revealed that things only started to improve when they decided to stop looking for other people to make them feel happy. They each took time to work on being happy themselves and came back together as stronger, more positive individuals. 'I needed to go away and gain my strength. Not as mummy; as myself.' These words from Jada stuck in my mind and helped me understand that having confidence really came down to having self-belief.

I realised that whilst having a support network is, of course, important, when it comes to building confidence or finding inner calm and contentment, we can't do any better than looking inside ourselves.

So how can I write a chapter on this when I'm not you? Well, let me start by saying that I'm actually not going to tell you how you can be confident. What I will share are insights into where you might start to find that self-belief and how we can all build on what's already there.

I'm a research geek. I love information and learning new skills and smooshing them together into one tasty sandwich. I know a little something about how postpartum feels too, having been on this journey three times now, but I'm also aware that, even as a seasoned mother, it doesn't make me the authority on all women's recovery.

So I've combined my personal experience with my professional expertise to bring you this chapter. I only wish I'd known it all in my twenties. Because the earlier we realise the power of supporting ourselves, the better!

Blunder and build

Feelings of confidence are tied in with our perception of our accomplishments and positivity towards our choices. The simple fact is that if we feel we've achieved something and done well, no matter how big or small the achievement, we're much more likely to put ourselves out there next time for another new challenge.

I read an article in which psychotherapist Amy Morin said, 'Healthy self-confidence is built by mastering new things and overcoming things you once thought you couldn't.'[29] In short, every time we acknowledge an achievement to ourselves, we're showing our brain that we are capable and stronger than we first thought.

There is a slight flaw in this plan, though. In order to achieve something, we must first have the confidence to try something, and that means we need to be willing to potentially fail. If we try and don't succeed, then what? Does that have the reverse effect? It turns out the answer to this is no, we don't actually have to succeed every time we try something in order to build confidence.

We've all heard the phrase 'That which does not kill us, makes us stronger', coined by philosopher Friedrich Nietzsche. But it's not just a sweet-sounding sentiment; there's truth behind it. Sometimes we need a blunder in order to begin building again, this time wiser and better prepared.

It's natural to feel uneasy about failure or embarrassment; however, according to experts we should instead view this as an opportunity to learn to deal with uncomfortable emotions, like disappointment. Every time we overcome a struggle we help ourselves learn to tolerate those uncomfortable feelings, giving us the confidence to try again.

This all highlights an uncomfortable truth, though: to build confidence we need to take action. We can't just think about something, say it and expect it to happen. The mantras we started with might help to move our mindset in the right direction, but sustaining that confidence is one step further.

Fuelling the flames of confidence

Interestingly, evolutionary psychologists believe that confidence is a key emotion that helped the human race survive.

In the days of our ancient ancestors, those with a strong sense of self-assurance would attract the most allies and be brave enough to explore further afield in order to get the resources needed for survival. By this reckoning, all of us alive today are descendants of the bravest and most confident people.

It is also believed that just like genetics, human behaviour can be passed down through generations too. So we all have it deep-rooted in our psyche to be confident. We just need to unearth this self-confidence and reconnect with it.

No emotion is stationary though, and confidence can fluctuate. We might be super confident in one area but fearful in another, so we could benefit from learning to transfer our confidence from stronger fields to other ones.

There have been plenty of times in my life where my self-confidence was low. As a young adult I started a career in the musical theatre industry, but after failing to recover from a vocal operation, I had to leave the industry that I had trained my whole life for. I had no idea what I was going to do next. To say my confidence was in tatters would be an understatement. I had to dig deep and figure out how to start on a new path. I wasn't confident, but I needed to find a way to build it back up.

To be honest, I think motherhood felt similar at first, although it was the catalyst for a huge confidence boost over time. After the birth of my first child, along with elation and excitement, I have a clear memory of looking down at the cot on the first night at home and thinking, So, *what now?* This was something I hadn't done before. I had no idea what I was doing; no book prepared me for this moment. I wasn't confident at all, but I needed to build it up quickly for the sake of my baby. To be honest, I still sometimes feel out of my depth with my eldest. Every day he gets older is a first for me as a mum.

I figured out right from those early days that I needed to throw myself in at the deep end and get stuff done. As the days went by, I realised that a lot of it did come naturally. It might not always have been the most graceful parenting style, but I was doing it and my son seemed happy, which I took as a good sign.

I realised something else as well. There can be some speed bumps that might trip us up on the road to self-assurance if we let them, but it can help a lot if we've prepared ourselves to cross them when they come.

❛INTERESTINGLY, EVOLUTIONARY PSYCHOLOGISTS BELIEVE THAT CONFIDENCE IS A KEY EMOTION THAT HELPED THE HUMAN RACE SURVIVE.❜

Speed bump tip number one: Nothing kills confidence like fear.

How fear functions

Fear is another human instinct passed down over millennia. Despite the feeling of discomfort it triggers in us, fear is crucial to survival. Historically, humans' ability to perceive a threat and recognise danger has kept us safe from predators, but in the modern world, with so many technological advancements and the demands placed on us day to day, whether these be financial, social or environmental, the opportunity for continued risk and long-term stress has increased and therefore fear has also.

When we set big goals, particularly ones we perceive as out of our reach, there will be a natural anticipation. We shouldn't invalidate those feelings, but we do need to push our boundaries a little. A thousand quotes come to mind: 'The best view comes after the hardest climb'; 'Nothing worth having ever came easy'; 'You have nothing to fear but fear itself'... But ultimately it's down to us; do we feel ready to test the waters and dip our toes in?

After acknowledging a fear, we should then rationalise it. What's the worst that can happen? We might encounter failure or a personal emotional battle, but our best armour is determination and persistence. Let's remember, even failing has its benefits.

Speed bump tip number two: Commitment is key!

Commitment

We might meet setbacks but we need to continue trying. We need to accept that at times we might fail, but we must make ourselves accountable for completing the task. Humans are hardwired to respect those who stick to what they say. More importantly *we* are hardwired to respect *ourselves* more if we stick to what we say! So, to build confidence we need to know that we will do what it takes to complete a task we set. Completing that action gives our words meaning.

At times it might feel hard. Sometimes we might even need to stop, regroup and try again. Days, weeks or months later. But progress is still progress, no matter how small.

I wish there was a way to sugarcoat all this, but then I'd be doing you a disservice.

Ultimately, you are actually in control of your confidence.

If you feel you're lacking confidence, ask yourself why. Your human nature and your instincts know that you are good enough, brave enough and capable enough. What is holding you back from believing in yourself?

FEAR IS ANOTHER HUMAN INSTINCT PASSED DOWN OVER MILLENNIA. DESPITE THE FEELING OF DISCOMFORT IT TRIGGERS IN US, FEAR IS CRUCIAL TO SURVIVAL.

Other people's perception

Some people might feel as though outside influence stops their confidence from growing. How others perceive us definitely can impact our confidence, but only if we allow it.

I've heard this from a lot of friends and first-time mums I've worked with. During a chat with Illiyin Morrison (@mixing_up_motherhood), who specialises in midwifery, I remember her saying, 'There's so much noise. Everyone has an opinion. It felt as though everyone was watching me and everyone could leave their review on what I was doing. Everyone was invested in how I did things.'

Many women are made to feel overwhelmed by other people's opinions and unsolicited advice on parenting, but another point Illiyin made stuck with me: 'At the end of the day, these people go home and don't think about us, yet we're left thinking about what they were saying.'

This resonated with me. During pregnancy I felt bombarded with messages from family, friends and even the media, about how motherhood 'should' be. Adverts telling me I just needed this one product to suddenly feel on top of the world.

But my true experience was nothing of the sort! Motherhood was liberating. I just needed to tap into how I truly felt and allow that to lead me.

Yes, there were days when things felt more challenging. But, on becoming a mum, I felt a lioness awaken. I found it the most animalistic and instinctive experience, once I let myself be free of the pressures of judgement.

At times, even as experienced mothers, we might find that we have absorbed stereotypes that others place on us. It happened after the birth of my twins. 'Twins are a different ball game,' I was told over and over, and I let myself believe it. Even though I had raised two children before, I found myself pushed into decisions, and the fear I felt about twins became overwhelming before they had even arrived.

Happily, the instant they were born this feeling melted away. It was a new experience for sure, but I looked at my children and knew we could do this. My confidence was back, and it was in the hands of two tiny twins. Together, I knew we were going to go about things in our own way and write our own story.

Yes, other people's opinions and stereotypes of what is 'right' can knock our confidence, so we should be aware of what we absorb from others. There is, however, another side to this coin. In the same way people bombarding us with their thoughts can be overwhelming, our confidence can also be knocked by someone's indifference. It can be difficult to be confident if you don't see others investing in you or believing in you.

I suppose what it comes down to is really accepting that we can't wait for someone else to lift us up. Just as I picked up from that Red Table talk, we need to believe in ourselves.

The social dilemma

It's understandable that we find ourselves in these confidence cycles, particularly with the rise of the virtual world. The influence that other people, brands and society have, telling us what we need in order to fit in, is accessible 24/7! It is strange that although 'likes' were originally created to spread positivity, they can now do more damage to our confidence than good.

A 'like' or 'follow' has become the highest form of bargaining chip. Watching others rocket to success in their career or 'bounce back' to their 'pre-baby body' can make us feel thoroughly depleted.

But the reality is that someone else's success doesn't impact ours.

The fitness industry can sometimes have this filter on it as though it's only for the athletic elite, but being body-confident doesn't mean you need to be body-'perfect'. We can be a work in progress and still be proud of ourselves. We are all works in progress.

When my eldest started school I told him over and over again to be proud of who he was, to always stay true to how he was feeling, and not be controlled by what others thought he needed to do to fit in. Well, let's put ourselves in the classroom, because we're practising exactly the same thing.

Looking on wistfully and comparing ourselves to others serves no purpose. Allowing ourselves to be steered by what others think serves no purpose. We need to let that go.

We're working on confidence and self-belief, and that is entirely down to ourselves.

Our bodies, our barriers and our self-belief

What came first, the chicken or the egg?

Well, physical wellbeing and confidence create a similar conundrum. Having a good relationship with one can boost the other. Exercise boosts our mood, and it's no secret that our mood also affects our ability and motivation to exercise.

During my dig into research on confidence and fitness, I came across a paper written by Daniel E. Lieberman, PhD. It was called 'Is exercise really medicine? An evolutionary perspective', and in this journal Lieberman wrote: 'Many lines of evidence indicate that humans evolved to be adapted for regular, moderate amounts of endurance physical activity into late age.'[30] Meaning, science is showing us that human beings are made to move, well into our senior years.

For our ancient ancestors, exercise was a necessity, but for modern humans it seems to be viewed more as a hobby. Even though we know there are health benefits, many people still lead fairly sedentary lives.

I could spend the next few pages listing all the benefits of exercise, in the hope of fanning the flames of confidence to get you started, but it's no secret that exercise is good for us and you can find the long list of reasons on any website, social site or blog platform – even on other pages within this book!

What fascinates me much more is how we need confidence to get moving in the first place. If human beings were born to move, what happened to break that instinctive chain in our minds?

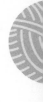

Confidence and exercise:
How to push past the fear

Perhaps you are hesitant about starting exercise because you experienced a birth trauma that has left you unsure of how to begin safely. Maybe you are reading this a few years after giving birth and worry it might be 'too late' to get started. Or perhaps you just haven't found the time and now feel out of practice. There can be many reasons that feelings of fear or nervous associations with exercise might develop.

If you feel this way, you are absolutely not alone. Research shows that up to 75 per cent of women feel the same and are worried about getting back into exercise.[31] Many want to be healthy but just don't have the confidence to get started.

So, how can we tackle that fear and overcome it?

Well, if starting to move your body just doesn't feel doable at first, then we can begin by moving our mind to a place where we then feel physically ready.

Here's an exercise that was recommended to me once to overcome a fear. I wanted to tackle a fear of heights. I had given birth twice at this stage and in the process had obliterated my fear of needles, and I was desperate to keep the momentum going. Anyone who's faced a fear and beaten it will know that the rush of achievement can be addictive!

After my fear of needles, heights were next on the list. It had crippled me for years and I'd missed so many fun opportunities because of it. The moment of facing this fear came at a bridge over a motorway.

I hated everything about this bridge. There was the height, obviously. The noise of the cars. The wind from any lorry that passed underneath.

The feeling that the rush of wind would just suck me under. The view from the middle where I just wanted to crouch down because each step felt like it would flip me on my head.

The funny thing is that I'd crossed this bridge plenty of times as a teenager without ever thinking, but in adulthood I had only ever crossed it once, whilst clinging on to my husband and the pram handle we were pushing. Afterwards I swore never to cross it again, nor put our child in such peril!

This bridge was right in the middle of my weekly run. I used to get there, stop, turn right around and run back, rather than cross over and complete the loop. I thought a few times about crossing but got a quarter of the way along and had to go back trembling.

My dad asked me, 'What would you say if a friend told you this? If they had this challenge that they really wanted to beat that was holding them back in their life. If they were missing out on things and they wanted to get better, but were scared. What would you say to them?' He suggested that I write down my response.

So I did. I put myself in the position of talking to a friend, and I started to put things into perspective. I realised then how much I had been missing out on and just how much this fear was ruining my confidence in other areas of my life. I was a mother, for goodness' sake. I could cross this bridge!

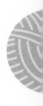

I tried a few more times ... and failed. But rather than give up and give myself a hard time, I imagined talking to this friend. I found I was much more compassionate and encouraging. I wrote down that failure was okay. I told my friend about everything that made her capable, all the things she'd done in the past that equipped her for this challenge. I told her that I believed in her, and told her how amazing she would feel once she'd done it. I told her no one fell off a bridge by getting swept up by the wind. I encouraged her not to give up, to keep trying, and that she should know her strength and one day she'd be confident enough to do it.

Then one morning I was at that bridge. I decided to not stop running. I didn't walk over or tip-toe to the edge like I usually would have. I didn't think too much, I just ran. I got halfway and felt sick. My running slowed right down and I realised I was halfway, my least favourite place, where I felt most vulnerable. I couldn't turn around. I knew if I stopped I literally might get stuck on this bridge. I didn't allow myself to focus on the fear I could feel rising within me. I thought of the empowering message I had written to my 'friend'. She was capable. Fear was just a figment of her imagination and I kept moving. Three more steps and I was over the halfway point. I could see the ground getting closer under my feet as I neared the other side.

I had done it! I turned around and ran straight back over. It was a moment of joy – or madness – because now I needed to go over again.

I noticed something else that day too. I felt much more confident when I had a choice than when I felt I 'had' to cross. Exercise can be similar. Nothing kills the fun of a workout like feeling you *have* to do it, rather than *want* to.

That said, sometimes we need to give ourselves a little push to get started, and right then I needed to push through that barrier and cross again. Which I did.

The exercise of talking to or writing to a friend allowed me to be compassionate with myself. I realised that by being so hard on myself for 'failure' in the past, I had been feeding my insecurities. I had been fueling myself with negative self-talk without even realising it.

When I got home, I took a few phrases from my letters. I wrote them out again and stuck them on a mirror. Even now I read them daily.

I ran over that bridge every week after that.

It's never too late. If you're reading this book five years after having children and have always avoided exercise because 'this is just you now', know that this mindset is a choice. You're the only thing in your way.

Few things feel as good as feeling capable, free and fearless.

If you have anxious thoughts about starting exercise or setting goals that just feel a little too out of your reach, write a letter to yourself as if you were talking to a friend. Show yourself some compassion and encouragement. Read that letter regularly! Fuel your mindset with confidence and care.

You deserve that. Don't give up.

❝ FEW THINGS FEEL AS GOOD AS FEELING CAPABLE, FREE AND FEARLESS. ❞

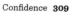

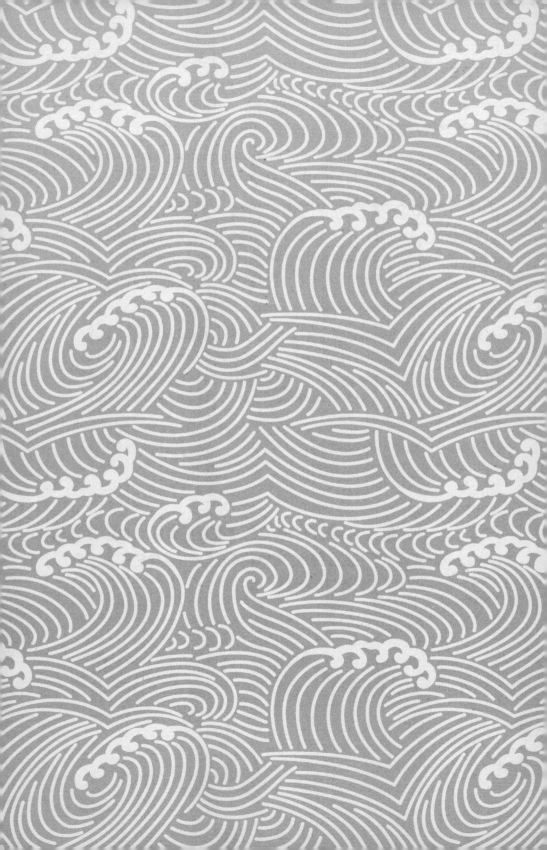

Motivation and maintenance

Motivation and maintenance . . . wow, those are some boring words, aren't they? Funny that the word motivation can sound so drab, but let me assure you, when we look into the psychology behind what motivates us, the subject is anything but dull.

Motivation and confidence, which we covered in the last chapter, can certainly go hand in hand, but as I began writing about the latter, I realised that I needed to give each its own space. Confidence we can build as we go, but motivation we want from the start!

Growing up, you could say I was surrounded by some fairly motivated individuals. My parents, for a start. My mum is an exercise recovery specialist and my dad an Olympic athlete turned motivational speaker. We used to travel abroad to California for my dad's athletics training during the summer, which meant that I also happened to be in the constant company of the Great Britain Athletics squad.

Okay, okay, fairly motivated was an understatement. I grew up with many incredibly inspiring examples of how hard work and motivation can pay off. I saw people demonstrating regularly, on and off the track, that if you believed you could, you would! Safe to say, it's inspired me my entire life.

Walter D Wintle's famous poem encompasses this perfectly:

> 'Life's battles don't always go
> To the stronger or faster man;
> But soon or late the man who wins
> Is the man who thinks he can.'

We know this to be true already from the section on affirmations in Chapter 2, where we saw how words and self-belief can impact our ability. But affirmations are just the beginning.

Skill, determination, time, effort and knowledge all play a part in achieving a goal. But feeling motivated is a big piece of the puzzle and one that many find difficult to fit.

Since becoming a mum, I find staying motivated comes with challenges different than in any other time in my life. The pressures of parenting and my strong desire to do it all right have sometimes meant that my exercise plan has had to take a back seat. If my children are unwell, for example, or are off school, my attention is diverted. I've had to find a way to stay committed to my goals, even when my plans change at the last minute. As mums we need to remain consistent with our intentions but flexible with our methods.

❛ AS MUMS, WE NEED TO REMAIN CONSISTENT WITH OUR INTENTIONS BUT FLEXIBLE WITH OUR METHODS. ❜

Inner or outer director?

First we need to distinguish between the two types of motivators that can fuel us. The first is the motivation that gets us started and the second is the motivation that keeps us going. The two work very differently. This is why, in my opinion, 'revenge body' motivation, where people fuel their fitness journey with ideas of flaunting their new figure in front of an ex, rarely works. The mad fury might kick you into action, but when you're looking for sustainable and positive change, this ain't gonna cut it.

We need to have a strong reason to keep focused that means more to us than 'revenge' on an ex. Something that can't be dismantled by anyone else's opinion, because ultimately, it's you who has to keep going. No one can support you better than you can support yourself.

It might seem daunting at first, the idea of going it alone, but actually it's incredibly powerful once you realise how capable you are. That's not to say we can't have a strong support network around us, but motivation is linked to our personal confidence, so we really do need to build self-belief.

We can often start by putting ourselves into one of two categories. We can be either 'inner-directed' or 'outer-directed'. Being 'inner-directed' means you are led by your own attitude and objectives, whilst 'outer-directed' people are impacted by their environment, circumstances and the people around them.

Every single one of us has a mixture of the two directives and their influence over us can fluctuate, depending on our mood or situation. There isn't a right or wrong way to be, but it does matter that we're aware of it, because it can affect how we choose to motivate ourselves.

In my teens and twenties I was a lot more outer-directed. I found the school environment encouraged feelings of comparison. In recent years, however, as I've grown up, and particularly since becoming a mother, I felt a definite shift. I wanted my children to grow up feeling confident and proud of who they are, not because someone else said it was okay but because they believed it themselves. And I realised I needed to model this for them.

Young children are actually often fantastic inner directors. The younger they are the more 'selfish' they seem to be, and I say that in awe not in judgement. Babies and toddlers do what they want to do. They aren't worried about how their actions might be perceived; they just act in a way that makes them happy. As we grow up, our experiences begin to shift how we think. We learn how to empathise and how our actions impact others. So on the one hand, being aware of our surroundings is important. But when we feel we need to look elsewhere to find encouragement or approval it has gone a step too far.

When it comes to sticking to a goal, finding inner-directed motivation is crucial. We need to root our decisions within our own beliefs. If we're continually looking at outside sources for instruction, it can prove tricky to sustain the motivation when the going gets tough.

Don't panic if you feel you might be outer-directed at the moment. As I said, many of us have a mixture of the two. I would encourage you to begin exploring your personal incentive, but for anyone who can't quite shake their outer director just yet, I'd recommend two things to stay motivated.

1 A workout buddy. Even if it's in a virtual sense, if you need others to keep a buzz going, connect with a community online or start a text chat with friends all about fitness goals to keep each other inspired.

2 State your aims. You're going to want to make yourself accountable by publicly stating your aims. You don't need to create a social media account to tell the world, but by letting those you trust know your intentions, you're already partially committing to the goal, which in itself is a great motivator. It's harder to give up once you've told people your mission.

Ultimately, an inner-directed goal will be best to keep us focused and grounded. Especially if we sometimes need to pause our workout plan because motherhood is calling, getting started again after time off can be one of the biggest challenges. An inner-directed goal can get us nicely back on track.

The other benefit of being driven from the inside is that, if someone questions our decision, we will know why we're doing it. We won't fold just because one person has made a snap judgement about our actions.

If you're stuck on finding a reason why, unfortunately I can't hand it to you because that would defeat the point of it being inner-directed, but perhaps it will help to start thinking about what exercise gives us. Aside from helping our physical recovery and soothing any aches, exercise can improve our mental health and can give us an energy boost. Plus with each workout completed, you'll experience the feeling of achievement, building confidence.

If you're still struggling, don't stress; read on and it might come to you. Maybe in finding your goal, your reason *why* will materialise!

Get that goal

Setting goals is a huge part of motivation. I never get as much out of a workout if I don't have at least a vague idea of what I'm going to do. If I'm honest, for a long time I thought 'goal-setting' was a little pretentious. Something reserved for people running marathons or for those with personal trainers who could guide them through the process. But as it turns out, we can all benefit from having something to work towards. Having a goal, no matter how small it might seem, can keep us focused and gives our actions purpose. Your goal doesn't have to be extreme, and, let me assure you, it's not a complicated process either.

SMART goals are a brilliant way to get going. SMART stands for Specific, Measurable, Achievable, Relevant and Time-bound.

The concept was originally started by two guys, Peter Ducker and George T. Doran in the 80s, who developed this method with regards to business management. But as time has gone on, this theory has been applied to many other areas of life, fitness being one of them.

We should consider all five points if we want to come up with a goal that can keep us focused and driven.

Think SMART

Specific. This is where our *why* comes in. The more specific we can be about what we want to accomplish and why, the easier it is for us to put steps in place to get there. Let's think about who else is involved (if at all), where our goal is set and what resources we need.

Measurable. Don't let this scare you; it's not an assessment you need to pass, but we do want a goal that we can measure. This will allow us to see our progress as it happens. 'I want to run', for example, is a little too vague, whereas 'I want to run for 10 minutes', or 'for 5km' gives us a much clearer direction. Then we can begin to plan our steps to get there.

It doesn't mean we should be judging ourselves every moment though; in fact, it's the opposite. Constant 'checking in' isn't productive and can lead to a negative addiction to exercise, or cause us anxiety. If we become obsessed with measuring our progress and testing ourselves too often, we will only notice small steps forwards which will feed feelings of frustration.

I'd recommend spacing out your progress checks in a similar way to how ultrasound scans during pregnancy are spread out across many months. When we're pregnant, the time between scans allows for substantial foetal development, and it's the same principle with ourselves postpartum. We need to allow time for change to take place. Postnatal recovery isn't a race – well, not if you want it to be sustainable at least!

I encourage you to think outside the box on how you measure your progress too. Often people assume that weight is the best indicator of health, but it's actually one of the least accurate ways to measure your fitness. The number you see on a scale has very little to do with your overall wellbeing, strength or even fat loss. In fact, it can often be that the more body fat we lose and the more muscle we create, the heavier we could weigh. This is because the fibres that form our muscles are compacted tighter together than those that make up body fat.

The compact design of our muscles means that we can fit more lean muscle fibres into a smaller space. Body fat, on the other hand, is more spaced out. It's lighter but takes up more room. It's like comparing a puffy cloud to concrete. High levels of body fat (clouds) could increase our dress size, even though we weigh less. When we exercise and continue to replace body fat with lean muscle (concrete), we can reduce in size but may actually weigh more.

Instead of weight, I recommend using physical challenges to test your progress. For example, I've been aiming to do five pull-ups, so every month I test how many I can do (currently at three-and-a-half)! We want the measure to be simple but informative. For example, you might monitor the number of push-ups you can do in a minute or how long you can jog for at a certain speed. Every 4 weeks is a good time frame to test your progress.

Achievable means making sure our goal is realistic. 'You can't shake your own shadow,' my dad used to say to me. What he meant was that I can't change who I am or where I'm starting from. I need to be realistic about where I am now. If you're not a marine biologist, no matter how much you want to deep-sea dive, planning to excavate a sunken treasure ship in 6 months probably isn't a realistic goal.

In the immediate postpartum period, this means accepting our current fitness level. This can be hard. I get it. The first time I gave birth, I had a swift recovery and within just a few months was almost back to my pre-pregnancy fitness condition. After my second and third births, however, things moved slower and I had distinct feelings of frustration.

Motivation and frustration are not a good match. One is constantly trying to keep you afloat whilst the other is attempting to pull you down.

Remember what Anna Mathur told me during our affirmation chat: that we should validate all our feelings. I knew that I couldn't ignore the frustration, but I couldn't wallow in it either.

We can acknowledge our frustration without letting it control us. We can combat those feelings by loving and supporting ourselves. Pregnancy, labour and birth are big achievements and they demand huge levels of physical strength from our body. Now it needs our support to get back to its regular rhythm.

That means acknowledging how it is feeling now, in the moment. As a general guideline I advise my clients to begin their postpartum exercise at the same intensity that they left their pregnancy fitness. For example, if you were performing press-ups on your knees at the end of your third trimester, I'd advise starting that way again.

When it comes to the big-picture goal, being realistic means we can lay strong foundations before progressing onwards.

Let me be totally clear: this doesn't mean thinking small. Being realistic is simply being honest with ourselves about where we're starting from and using that to plan properly how we're going to get where we want to go.

Relevant. Making our goal relevant helps us to stay committed. If you can answer yes to questions like, 'Is it worthwhile?'; 'Can you make the time?'; and 'Is it a positive influence in your life?', then that's a great indicator of a goal that matters. A goal that is too abstract – like excavating the sunken treasure ship – might cause us more stress than pleasure. That's not to say we can't be creative with what we want to achieve. If you want to run 10km but feel like a total novice, that's still a very realistic goal. We just need a goal that we can line up to some degree with our lifestyle and environment.

Time-bound. Don't let this make you nervous. Setting a time frame for your goal is paramount to staying focused. It doesn't need to be done in a few weeks. Maybe we're looking at a monthly or yearly target. What is important is that alongside our 'big goal' we need to have smaller checkpoints along the way too.

Just like ticking off landmarks on the way to a holiday, we can have exercise landmarks, so that we can see the journey we're on is paying off and we're getting closer to our final destination.

When I was a child my family would drive to Germany to visit my grandparents. For six-year-old me, the prospect of such a long drive felt tedious and almost unachievable. To keep us entertained and to avoid the repeated 'Are we there yet?' chorus, my mum suggested we tick off places that we recognised on a list. Every time we drove there it was the same: we ticked off our favourite places to indicate that we were closer to our grandparents, and closer to the celebratory welcome cake (thank you, German traditions!).

The Channel Tunnel, the Belgian border, the Warburg arches – all of them let us know we were getting closer and closer. I would literally feel the excitement building. It's the same as we get closer to a fitness goal.

Feel that excitement as you tick off your landmark list: 1km, five press-ups, two lengths ... Allow those achievements to motivate you more. Acknowledge these mini-successes, and celebrate your arrival at each one.

In reality

There's one final consideration that's needed for setting a good goal. And it's pretty much non-negotiable for us mums. That is the ability to be flexible with all of the above!

Not reaching your goal in the set time frame isn't failure. It's life. I have lost count of the number of times that I made plans, set goals or had deadlines, only to realise that my children don't actually care about my schedule. Sometimes. as parents, we just need to roll with the moment.

Goal-setting is great to make sure we have clear intentions, but if we need extra time to complete the goal, then let's give ourselves that space without also giving ourselves a hard time for it.

Positive or negative addiction to exercise

I mentioned that putting too much pressure on ourselves to achieve a goal can lead to feelings of anxiety or a negative addiction to exercise. I remember when I first read about positive and negative addictions to exercise. The concept was interesting to me because I hadn't ever considered exercise as a negative before, but as with all things, I suppose, too much of a good thing isn't great either.

Exercise should leave us feeling positive and energised. It should be something we look forward to but aren't completely obsessed with or controlled by. Signs of shifting into a negative addiction can be finishing a workout but still feeling drained or irritated, or you might find that the idea of missing a workout causes stress. That's not to say all workouts will have us on cloud nine, but we should be feeling good about getting moving.

If you feel you might be negatively addicted to exercise, it's already a good step that you can recognise it. Take a few steps back and look at your 'why'. It can be easy to get lost in the desire to improve quickly, but let's remember why we're really here and all the many other benefits that come with leading a healthy lifestyle. Exercise is meant to support your body and mind, not deplete them.

We can feel physically tired at the end of a workout, without being drained. We can't escape the fact that exercise takes effort. We will need to drive forwards with our goals, but always keep an eye on how our mood and mindset are affected.

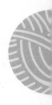

The role of rest

Whilst we're talking about achieving goals, I think it's a good idea to make it clear that rest is a part of that process. We've touched on the role of rest before in Chapter 11. And with so much evidence supporting the fact that humans need rest in order to survive, it's strange that sometimes, it is seen as synonymous with being lazy. That couldn't be further from the truth. In fact, when it comes to exercise, our bodies use the down time during rest to reap the full benefits from a workout.

Did you know that placing extra demands on your body when it's already under stress can actually work against a weight-loss goal?

I remember listening to Clare Goodwin (@thepcosnutritionist) speaking at a wellbeing festival a few years ago about just this topic. She mentioned that in her twenties, as a professional triathlete competing for New Zealand, she encountered a crossroads, where she was exercising at extremely high levels but somehow still finding that her body fat stores were increasing and she was gaining weight. It turns out that these high levels of exercise were actually the cause! 'Over-exercising is a form of stress,' Clare told me. 'And sometimes, it can be that high stress levels for the body or the mind can cause weight gain.'

❝DID YOU KNOW THAT PLACING EXTRA DEMANDS ON YOUR BODY WHEN IT'S ALREADY UNDER STRESS CAN ACTUALLY WORK AGAINST A WEIGHT-LOSS GOAL?❞

To give you the facts in a nutshell, stress can trigger the release of the hormone cortisol into our body. In Chapter 8, we touched on how our primal animal instincts are programmed to interpret this rise in stress as a sign that there must be some kind of threat, which causes the release of glucose (simple sugars) into our system. Our body can use this energy to flee from or confront the danger (fight or flight). However, in modern life, stress isn't only triggered by a physical threat. We might feel stress from work pressures or relationship issues or the increased demands of early parenthood.

In these cases, we might be sat at our desk unable to flee, so we aren't physically expending the energy. Our body isn't using the glucose so it then stores this as body fat. If we then place extra stress onto our body, by upping the physical demands e.g. adding more workouts, the body will produce even more glucose and therefore begin to store more body fat.

If this continues for a long time, it could cause our body to become resistant to the hormone called insulin. Insulin's main role is to help our cells use glucose for energy. If we become resistant our body will struggle even more to use body fat as energy and instead begins to break down our own muscle mass.

So rest isn't 'lazy'; it's crucial! Rest and relaxation will reduce our cortisol levels. If you're feeling drained or overwhelmed, make sure you also prioritise mindfulness, meditation or straight up sleep, alongside your exercise. Adaquate rest can help to manage your blood sugar levels, allowing your body to function more efficiently.

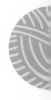

Maintaining our motivation

Now we've found our motivation, it's a different ball game to maintain it. Here are some quick tips to keep that fire burning!

1 Plan ahead

I don't mean a weekly workout schedule; we've established that flexibility is key. I mean a session plan. If I start a workout and have no clue what exercises I'll include, ultimately it ends up an uncoordinated and unproductive mess. I'll probably do a few squats, press-ups and planks, and then my imagination wears thin. Nowadays, with multiple social media platforms (like mine, hint hint), you have unlimited access to great workouts specifically designed for pre- and postnatal women, but you can also go old-school and just write down a few moves of your own.

For the immediate postnatal period Chapter 10 has quite a few to choose from, and once you're ready to up the intensity, head on over to Chapter 15 for lots of exercise progressions!

2 Small acts of commitment

Simple steps that commit you to your plan can make all the difference between getting a workout done and not finding the time. Laying out your gym clothes the night before, for example. It's uncomplicated but effective. If we're dressed and ready, we save time and are instantly put in the mindset to get moving. As a mum, I invested in some quality nursing sports bras too (they do exist!) and I pretty much lived in them.

We can prepare our food too. If you head over to StrongLikeMum.com you'll find a ton of options for nutritious and quick snacks and lots of food we can cook ahead of time to use when our days are jam-packed.

After my first son was born, I lost count of the times I would return from a jog and barely have time to shower before he needed feeding, changing or entertaining. Somehow the freezer would be full of pre-cooked baby purées, but never a nutritious snack for myself. I made sure to plan ahead the next time.

3 Playlist or podcast?

Music equals motivation! Am I right? Well, it turns out that half of you reading this will think I'm wrong! I was convinced everyone felt like me, that you need good beats to boost motivation, but apparently it depends on who you ask. I was sitting with a group of friends recently and the debate broke out between whether people preferred listening to music or talking during exercise, and the result was pretty much an even split. Only a few said they'd rather not listen to anything. (I know, I don't get this either!)

Personally, I listen to music whenever I need to get focused. In fact, I listened to music during all of my births too. I found it was great to keep my energy up and anxiety down. In my caesarean I even took a tip from a friend Sarah (@disasterofathirtysomething) and sang my way through it!

I don't need to tell you that music can trigger emotional responses. We've all belted out that number-one tune in the car or sobbed into our pillow during a sombre ballad. It's undeniable, music touches our soul. And, believe it or not, it has actually been shown to improve physical performance too. Studies have found that music can lead to us having higher endurance levels, increased strength and a marked improvement in our work capacity![32] So whether you're listening to spiritual awakenings from Enya, indulging in Pavarotti, or busting beats from the latest chart-toppers, get your playlist lined up because it's definitely going to help you stay focused!

That's not to say a decent podcast doesn't have its place. I'm all for learning a little something, especially when I'm out for longer runs. I might still need a strong beat to get my butt up a hill, but switch back to a podcast for distraction as I chalk up the kilometres. Whatever you choose, audio stimulation is great for maintaining motivation.

4 Enjoy it!

Music might help your exercise become just that, enjoyable! But we can do other things to make the movement more fun too. Not all fitness fans need to be gym-goers or yoga experts, there's a whole beautiful world in between. Traditional exercises like push-ups or squats are just one way to keep active. Once your core rehab is in place, don't be afraid to try a variety of exercise, whether that's dancing around the living room, going for a kayak or taking a hike. It's good to challenge our body in new ways, and getting active in any way you enjoy is key to sustaining a drive!

5 Find the time of day that works best for you

I've read countless studies on when is best to work out. Some people are adamant that early morning workouts yield the best results, whilst others rate a pre-dinner session as their preferred choice. There's research supporting both: some studies have suggested that exercising first thing, before breaking your fast, is ideal if you have a fat-burning goal, provided you refuel properly afterwards. An afternoon session might see you benefitting from extra energy for the remainder of the day, and an evening session is thought to prime your body for better sleep along with other benefits. The options seem endless!

For us mums, I think we need to set our own rules. Call me crazy but I believe that the best experts to decide when would be a good time to work out is us!

I always ask myself these questions:

1 When do I have the most energy?
2 When will my children be happy to occupy themselves for a while?

Fitting in a workout when you have a family is not simply about finding the time to move; it's making sure that everyone else is ready for us to exercise too. At least that's my experience.

My kids are usually in a better mood in the morning. So if I can't get out before they wake up, then I use the twins' first nap of the day to exercise, 1–3 times a week. Whilst the babies sleep, the older children are usually happy to play, or relax, and if anyone does wake up mid-session they're often happy to sit and watch for a while.

In short, identify what time of the day seems best for your family and aim to exercise then.

6 Get yourself a workout buddy

People are much less likely to give up on a commitment to a partner than they are to themselves. Even if face-to-face get-togethers don't happen often, making a commitment to a workout partner and regularly keeping in touch will keep you on track.

I gave birth to my twins during the UK lockdown in 2020, and the government restrictions meant I couldn't leave home to exercise with friends at all. What I could do, though, was set up a text group. A few friends and I would share our postnatal journey and exercise achievements. It became a fabulous support network for my physical and mental health.

7 Wanderlust workouts

Look at your schedule on a week-by-week basis. That was what felt achievable to me. Looking any further ahead seemed impossible: by the end of the month so many unforeseen things would have popped up that there was no point in planning so far in advance. Any less than a week and I would feel frustrated about not knowing whether I'd have another space of time to myself. So, on Sunday evenings my husband and I would spend 5 minutes saying when we would like to work out that coming week. We ended up calling these our 'wanderlust workouts'. Wanderlust is a German phrase, meaning 'a desire to travel', because, somehow, no matter what we agreed, these workouts would often move from where we'd put them! They'd wander about to different times and different days entirely. Such is family life, hey, always unpredictable!

You might wonder then, what the point is in scheduling workouts if we know their times might change, but somehow having a rough idea of what the other person was planning allowed us to manage our expectations and help support each other's goals when we could.

Here's a rough example:

To begin with, highlight two times a week you'd like to fit in a workout (*) and a third time which acts as a backup if you can (^).

Make sure to allow for a rest day between each workout, or if you have more than three sessions, that you have no more than two consecutive workout days.

Mon	Tues	Wed	Thurs	Fri	Sat	Sun
*	R	R	*	R	^	R

On rest days it's important that our body is able to recover and consolidate the effects of our previous workout. If you're worried that a day off might lead you to 'fall off the wagon', you can use your rest days to stretch, read something about health and wellbeing or experiment with a new recipe. This will support us in staying connected to our goals and encourage a healthy outlook on our overall lifestyle.

On the days when you do work out, plan roughly six exercises to fill a half-hour session – that's allowing for two repetitions of each exercise, if they last between 30 and 40 seconds. Of course, the time will change depending on whether you need to repeat anything on the other side and how much rest you take between each movement, but as a basic outline it works. If you're just starting out you might want to begin with 20 seconds of each exercise, followed by 15 seconds of rest, progressing to 30 seconds of work and 15 of rest once you're ready.

Finally, have an idea of where you'd like to work out – the garden, living room or gym, for example. Note down if you'll be needing any equipment or if there's a commuting time to another location, like the gym or a park run.

❛LOOK AT YOUR SCHEDULE ON A WEEK-BY-WEEK BASIS. THAT WAS WHAT FELT ACHIEVABLE TO ME.❜

Choosing exercises

Each stage of postpartum recovery has a different focus. We've covered this in detail in Chapters 8 through 15 but here's a quick refresh for any of you who might have been half-asleep when you read that!

Weeks 0–6 are focused on engaging our deep core, harnessing the connection between our mind and body, and mobilising our joints and ligaments again post-birth.

Weeks 6–12, once cleared for exercise by a medical professional, you can begin to up the intensity of your workouts. Initially we still want to keep the impact low. Our body will continue to have lots of perinatal hormones fluctuating throughout its system, so we don't want to over-stress our joints or ligaments. These next few weeks will involve a whole-body approach, which means that we target the entire body during each movement, as opposed to isolating the upper or lower body. The focus is on re-engaging with exercise, further rehabilitation of our core and building strong foundations.

Weeks 12–24 are when we can up the intensity and begin to incorporate impact exercises safely. This is a general timeline; every woman is, of course, different, and your medical team might advise you to wait a little longer. Always follow their advice as they can give you a one-to-one, hands-on assessment, which is tricky through the pages of a book!

Let this time be a celebration of what your body has achieved and use that to inspire you to make a commitment to yourself. Using exercise, nutrition and a healthy lifestyle, we can help our bodies progress on the road to recovery at a time that works for us.

Weeks 24 and beyond means we reached the 6-month postpartum mark. Hopefully our little newborns are giving us a tad more sleep at night, and, with weaning beginning around now, we may be freed up a little more, occasionally leaving our children with family or close friends to get a little solo time.

By now we will ideally have been able to incorporate more functional exercises into our training programme, having moved our core work off the floor, and activating our support network during movements. We can slowly increase the intensity of our workouts and switch our mindset to maintaining our progress.

Some people might find this time one of the trickiest mentally when it comes to exercise. After the birth of my twins, I remember reaching 6 months postpartum and feeling really frustrated that I wasn't further along with my fitness level. I had to remind myself that although 6 months felt like a long time and things were beginning to settle down, I was still a long way off full recovery. Many experts are adamant that it can take up to 18 months for your body to completely recover after pregnancy, so although 6 months feels like a long time, it's very early in the scheme of things.

To make sure we don't overexert ourselves, let's remember the signs of a negative addiction to exercise we just discussed, as well as the red flags outlined in Chapter 5 (see page 78).

Slow recovery shouldn't be demoralising. If anything, let's challenge that mindset and remember that by taking our time we are actually laying strong foundations in our core that can give our body the best support to be more powerful, strong and stable in the future.

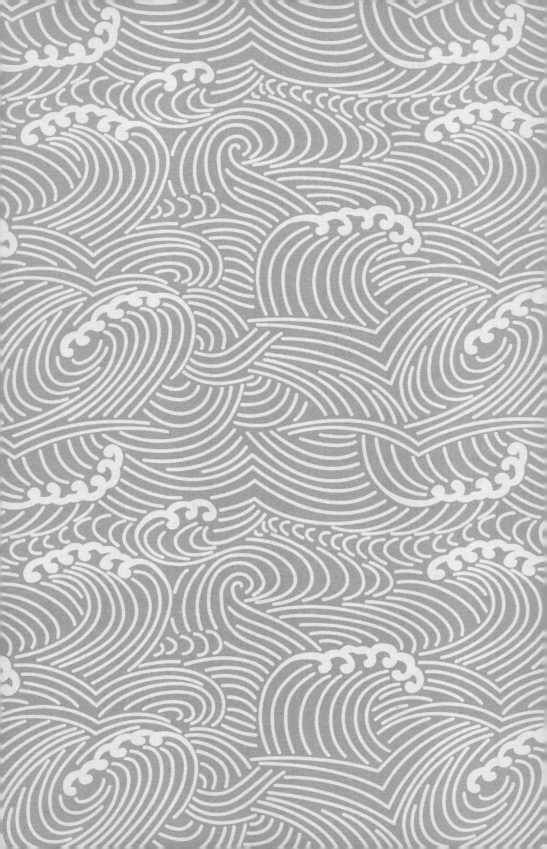

Myth-busting for mamas

I started out creating StrongLikeMum to shatter the stereotypes surrounding pre- and postnatal health. I wanted to break down the barriers to any questions women felt unsure about or afraid to ask for fear of being judged.

I asked a million questions during my pregnancies, and I've also been fortunate enough to work in this industry for a decade, meeting wonderful women and experts who have enabled me to learn new information all the time.

I've taken many, many notes over the years and I'm happy to share the answers I've found here, all of which are backed up by studies, professional expertise and personal experience.

Prenatal questions

Can pregnancy affect vision?

This was new to me when I first heard it, but after extensive research it turns out that this is, in fact, true. Ocular changes such as blurred vision affect approximately 15 per cent of pregnant women.[33]

There are several ways your vision might be affected during pregnancy, which experts believe are usually due to our hormones. One such change could be that there is a decrease in tear production (which is ironic as pregnancy hormones are stereotypically attributed to making us more emotional and teary). But this dryness can irritate our eyes and cause discomfort.

To completely contradict the above, some women actually find that they suffer a build-up of fluid in their eyes, similar to the water build-up around our ankles and feet. Experts believe that this pressure could change the curvature of the eye, making it more sensitive.

Other changes in vision could include a decrease in peripheral vision or a thickening of the cornea.

As is often the case with pregnancy and postpartum, everyone reacts differently and whilst some women notice a change in their vision, many experience no change at all.

If you experience this it can sound daunting and worrying; however, research has shown that changes to eyesight will return to normal postpartum. You should seek the advice of a medical professional if you experience changes to your vision.

What is prenatal saliva increase and will I need a spit cup?

Ahhhh, the spit cup, which is every bit as disgusting as it sounds. It's quite literally a cup of saliva!

You may be nodding in agreement here, or perhaps you're wondering what on earth this unappetising image has to do with pregnancy. Well, for some pregnant women, and I was one of them, carrying around a cup of yuk can be necessary due to the increased production of saliva during pregnancy. And, yep, you guessed it, we can blame our hormones again!

The nerves that control salivation are more stimulated than usual when we are pregnant, leading to this over-production, called ptyalism. For many this can ease after the first trimester; however, for a few it can last the entire pregnancy. This increase in saliva has no harmful effects to baby, but the bitter taste and mucous sensation may increase feelings of nausea which can be upsetting or uncomfortable for the mother.

When can I start exercising if I'm a beginner?

Many women feel afraid to start exercise during pregnancy if they weren't used to working out before. But, not only is getting active beneficial for mum and baby, it's actually recommended as a great way to enjoy a happy and healthy pregnancy!

How much exercise should I do?

Currently it's recommended that pregnant women should aim for approximately 150 minutes of moderate-intensity aerobic activity every week, with a minimum of 3 x 15-minute sessions for those who led a sedentary lifestyle pre-pregnancy.[34]

You may have heard that pregnancy is not the time to try something new, but this is not necessarily the case. Starting an active lifestyle can be perfectly safe. After all, if pregnancy is the first time you're starting to exercise then everything will be new.

It is true, however, that pregnancy is not the time to begin pushing your physical boundaries to extremes. Running, for example, is only recommended if you have previous experience with the sport.
As an alternative, lacing up for a walk and some gentle body-weight movements is great provided you have been cleared for exercise by a medical professional and are experiencing an uncomplicated pregnancy.

Does pregnancy cause a change in skin tone?

Although it's not spoken about much, many women experience a change in their skin colour during pregnancy. It's common for women to develop patches of darker skin. This condition is known as melasma or chloasma and is more likely to affect women with darker complexions. The changes in skin pigmentation most commonly disappear on their own after delivery.

Often referred to as 'the mask of pregnancy', this change may lead to differences of pigmentation on a woman's face, and skin that is already pigmented, such as nipples and scars. The skin around your genitals may also become darker.

The most recognised change in skin pigmentation is the darkening of the linea negra, a line running vertically down the middle of the abdomen, which is a form of hyperpigmentation often seen in pregnant women.

Postnatal questions

What are postnatal hot sweats?

Approximately 35 per cent of women experience night sweats in pregnancy and just under 30 per cent postpartum.[35] We can thank our lovely hormones again.

Partly due to the decreasing levels of progesterone and oestrogen, night sweats (or hot sweats) may also occur due to excess water retention which some women develop in pregnancy. All the extra fluid the body took on to support the pregnancy is now looking for a way out, so sweating and urination may increase initially as a way to flush the fluids out.

To help you cope, wear loose-fitting clothing when possible, make sure to stay hydrated and have a spare set of bedsheets ready if you need a quick change in the night! Exercise and nutrition can also help by assisting with an efficient recovery and supporting overall better sleep.

Night sweats should ease after the first few weeks postpartum. If symptoms continue after your 6–8 week check, it's advised to run it by your doctors who can investigate more.

❝CURRENTLY IT'S RECOMMENDED THAT PREGNANT WOMEN SHOULD GET APPROXIMATELY 150 MINUTES OF MODERATE-INTENSITY AEROBIC ACTIVITY EVERY WEEK...❞

Is breastfeeding painful?

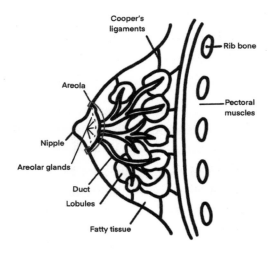

Cooper's ligaments

Rib bone

Areola

Pectoral muscles

Nipple

Areolar glands

Duct

Lobules

Fatty tissue

I didn't fully understand the importance of 'latch' until my second son was born. My first experience of breastfeeding had been physically an 'easy' one. But after my second son was born, I experienced the challenges other women had told me about.

Having a good latch can make all the difference between comfortable and difficult breastfeeding. Your baby will be feeding every 2–3 hours in the early days, so any unresolved issues can worsen quickly if not amended. Your baby should be drawing in a large portion of the lower part of your areola (the dark circle around your nipple) when feeding with your nipple positioned against the roof of their mouth, supported by their tongue. If you feel you may be struggling with your latch, or experience any sustained pain when nursing, speak with your midwife, lactation consultant or other healthcare providers for further advice. There are often good breastfeeding support networks available for new mums. Don't be fooled into thinking that because breastfeeding is an instinctive act, it will instantly be a piece of cake!

Facing a challenge with breastfeeding is surprisingly common, with one survey suggesting that over 90 per cent of women face breastfeeding challenges within the first three days.[36] Fortunately the majority of these issues can be solved with simple guidelines.

During the first few days after birth, your breasts will produce colostrum, the first type of nutritional milk your body produces. It has a sticky consistency and is yellowy-orange in colour. After three to four days your breastmilk will 'come in'. This process can cause some discomfort at first as your breasts become enlarged to accommodate the increased milk supply, but this should settle down after the first few feeds.

Some women worry about feeling pain from breastfeeding. When the latch is good, breastfeeding is not painful; however, it can often be uncomfortable if the latch isn't quite right. Some women also report a short sensation of discomfort, for the first few seconds when baby latches on and draws the breast into its mouth. This should cease quickly if a good latch is achieved. You may also experience discomfort if your nipples become sore, cracked or blistered. Nipple salve can be a good barrier and treatment for sore nipples, and shouldn't interfere with baby's feeding.

Breast shields can also be used to prevent rubbing from clothing. Some women may choose to use breast shields during feeding as a barrier for sore nipples, but you should discuss this option with a lactation specialist first.

Women should also be encouraged to try different breastfeeding positions. There are various positions to breastfeed in, for example a cradle hold, underarm 'rugby ball' or lying-down position. It's worth trying a variety of positions to see how you feel most comfortable.

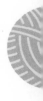

What is lactation mastitis?

This is a condition which causes inflammation of the breast tissue, causing breast pain, swelling or redness. It's believed this occurs either by a blocked milk duct or by bacteria entering your breast. Sometimes this can resolve on its own; however, always check symptoms with your doctor who may refer you for further treatment.

If you are able to manage your mastitis at home, a warm damp towel may help to relieve pain, in addition to breast massage, hand expressing or frequent feeding (if you can bear it) to relieve a blocked duct. You should also prioritise rest and staying hydrated.

Some women have even suggested that chilled dry green cabbage leaves help with pain. In this case, be sure to cut out a gap for your nipple in the middle but cover the rest of your breast.

If needed, some over-the-counter pain medications are considered safe for breastfeeding mothers and can help with pain management.

Any other breastfeeding tips?

'Let down' is the term given to the sudden release of milk from your breast. This is a normal reflex for many women and occurs when the nerves in our breast become stimulated. This can be due to your baby latching on, but it can also be triggered emotionally, such as by hearing a baby cry.

Let down can sometimes take us mums by surprise, so many women choose to place breast pads over their nipples to prevent leaking through their clothes. In this case, make sure to replace your breast pads regularly if required.

Whilst breast pads themselves won't cause mastitis, infrequent changing of pads may. Bacterial growth is the biggest potential risk and leading cause of mastitis. Bacteria thrive in warm and moist environments so changing your pads regularly to keep the area clean is important.

How can I manage stretch marks?

Stretch marks are a result of our skin stretching quickly. They can develop in the later stages of pregnancy. Some women never have a single stretch mark, whilst others find that they develop many. Early stretch marks can be red, purple or pink in appearance and feel slightly raised or itchy, but with time the colour fades and the narrow bands sink back beneath your skin.

Stretch marks are permanent; however, not only do they reduce in appearance over time, but treatments may help to alleviate the itch and make them less noticeable.

Simple measures such as applying moisturiser or a gel have been shown to have some effect on reducing the signs of stretch marks. However, any treatment you try should always be checked with a medical professional. What does seem to be agreed is that applying your ointment to stretch marks early is important to improving the overall appearance.

Staying well hydrated in pregnancy could also play a part in preventing stretch marks or reduce the number of stretch marks someone develops. Hydrated and soft skin is more flexible and as such may not scar as easily as dry skin.

How can I manage postnatal incontinence?

Suffering with urinary incontinence post-birth can be very common, but this doesn't need to be your 'new normal'.

During pregnancy, as baby grows and hormonal changes take place, more pressure is placed on your bladder and pelvic floor muscles. The joints and ligaments in this area are also loosened. Regardless of whether you give birth vaginally or via a caesarean section, you may experience some level of urinary incontinence postpartum. This may cause leaking when you lift something heavy, cough, sneeze, laugh or exercise.

Discreet incontinence pads can be used to absorb urine loss. However, this is a short-term solution, and exercise of the deep core and pelvic floor can be used to help alleviate symptoms. Exploring the pelvic floor exercises outlined in this book, such as those indicated in Chapter 9 and Chapter 15, can help us to see marked improvements.

Let's remember that it's not just a weak pelvic floor that could be the cause of incontinence. An overactive (over-tight) pelvic floor can sometimes also cause urinary incontinence and other uncomfortable symptoms such as difficulty urinating, the urge to empty your bladder frequently, pain during sexual intercourse or lower back ache. If you think this might apply to you, relaxation techniques for the pelvic floor like those on page 59, and jaw and feet relaxation on page 166, may be better suited to your recovery.

If you have persisting symptoms of urinary incontinence, reach out to your GP or wider medical team for further investigation.

Faecal incontinence may also occur postpartum, affecting up to 5 per cent of women. This is often due to damage of the anal sphincter during childbirth. Your medical team will discuss treatment options with you that will be suitable to your individual experience.

Other lifestyle factors including diet and hydration can also play a role in pelvic floor health. Caffeine is known to irritate your pelvic floor and bladder so limit consumption if you can.

Also try to avoid nicotine if possible. Smoking has been shown to affect the lining of the bladder. Chronic coughing, sometimes caused by smoking, can also increase stress and pressure on your bladder and pelvic floor.

If symptoms of any incontinence persist, speak with your GP who may refer you to a women's health physio.

What's a Kegel and am I doing them right?

Whilst we don't want to overtrain our pelvic floor, Kegel exercises do have fantastic benefits and can be really useful as part of our overall training programme.

In this book we've covered quite a few pelvic floor exercises that work on engaging and strengthening this muscle group. All of them are a form of Kegel exercise.

A Kegel exercise is simply a contraction of the pelvic floor muscles. The name 'Kegel' came from Dr Arnold H. Kegel, an American gynaecologist who developed these exercises in the late 1940s as a nonsurgical way to prevent women from leaking urine.

As described in the exercises throughout this book, to fully engage your pelvic floor muscles you need to visualise your coccyx bone (at the back) and pubic bone (at the front) coming together and lifting up. You might have heard trainers encouraging people to 'imagine you're stopping the flow of urine', 'imagine you're trying to avoid passing gas' or 'tighten your vagina around a tampon'. I find these visualisations are not as effective at encouraging complete pelvic floor activation, but they are, in essence, trying to get the client to do the same thing.

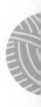

How long do I need to wait before engaging in sexual intercourse?

A midwife once told me that she'd known a couple to have intercourse at the hospital within just 24 hours of giving birth. Well, I simply can't fathom how! Sex after giving birth was almost as scary to me as that first postpartum poop. I knew it would happen sometime, but I had no idea how it would feel. Would there be repercussions after giving birth?

If you feel as I did, and are a little nervous about how things will feel, here are the facts.

It is advised to wait at least 2 weeks before engaging in sex postpartum. Having intercourse too early increases the risk of postpartum haemorrhage or uterine infection. Many medical professionals may even advise waiting for your 6–8 week check. This will greatly depend on your personal recovery. As with postnatal exercise, what's crucial is that you feel ready. There are no strict statistics on when you'll be ready for sex post-birth, but the previous guidelines give a rough idea.

Many women may also find that they experience vaginal dryness in the early postnatal days, which can be due to low oestrogen levels. This can last a few weeks or for breastfeeding women possibly longer. It's also been suggested that breastfeeding may temporarily reduce a woman's sex drive.

Once you do feel ready for sex, just make sure that your pelvic floor has recovered and that the postpartum lochia (postpartum bleeding) has stopped.

What is the caesarean pouch and will it settle down?

The caesarean pouch, or 'c-shelf', can come as a bit of a shock for some women. I certainly wasn't expecting it myself. The scar I knew about, but not a pouch of loose skin! However, since my caesarean, I've been hard pressed to find a woman who hasn't had one, whether temporarily or long-term.

This can be difficult to come to terms with and may seem overwhelming to start with, but time can do wonders for recovery, post-caesarean pouch included. I noticed a huge improvement of my incision site after the first year postpartum.

How your personal recovery will be depends on many things. As always, we need to appreciate that all women are unique.

The post-caesarean pouch is thought to be a combination of post-surgery swelling, loose skin and excess fat.

During a caesarean birth, the surgeon will cut into multiple layers, firstly skin followed by subcutaneous fat and then deeper fascia, which covers our muscles and organs. After delivery, each layer will be closed back up, first with the uterus and then working outwards.

The development of scar tissue is inevitable after any incision. Scar tissue is thought to only ever reach about 70 per cent of the strength of the tissue it has replaced, but it can feel tough or even rubbery to touch. Over time scar tissue can soften and eventually become less pronounced. The best way to facilitate this is with mobilisation massage techniques as outlined on page 154.

The swelling we notice in this area after surgery is a natural response by the body as it begins healing itself. As part of the recovery process, thousands of cells are sent to the affected body part. This is part of the first stage of healing and is referred to as the inflammatory phase. This will settle down within a few weeks and we will notice a marked difference.

The elasticity of our skin will also play a role in the aesthetic appearance of our caesarean incision site. Part of our skin's make-up will be genetic and is something we have little control over; however, staying hydrated and moisturising our skin during pregnancy can improve the elasticity of our skin to some degree. This is not, however, to suggest that any creams will get rid of your caesarean pouch, so don't be hoodwinked by flashy adverts telling you the opposite!

This is because a big part of the caesarean pouch is down to the layer of subcutaneous fat, which lies underneath our skin. Although this layer of fat is visible under the skin, it's usually harmless and may even protect us against some diseases. It's visceral fat that surrounds our organs on a much deeper level that has been associated with various health diseases.

A healthy diet and regular exercise can help us to manage the levels of fat in our body. Postnatal-specific core exercises can also help us manage the appearance of our tummy postpartum. However, this should be a slow and controlled process.

So, is it possible to get rid of the postpartum pouch?

Well, as you can see, there is no straightforward answer. Every woman heals differently. We can certainly make marked improvements to the appearance of our incision site, but to varying degrees there will undoubtedly be evidence of our caesarean birth.

Coming to terms with this may be challenging, particularly if the caesarean was unplanned. If you feel as though you are struggling, you can request a birth debrief to understand more about your delivery and communicate how you are feeling. You may also wish to explore other options with your GP, whether in an emotional support capacity or further treatment options such as referral to a women's health physio or surgical intervention specialist.

What about postnatal hair loss?

First things first: don't panic. If you experience postpartum hair loss, know that the effects of this are usually temporary, plus, as many women retain more hair during pregnancy, the postnatal loss can at times be barely noticeable.

On average we shed about fifty to one hundred hairs every day, when we're not considered pre- or postnatal. During pregnancy this number is lower, mainly due to hormones like the rising levels of oestrogen, which encourages our hair to sustain the growth phase of our hair-growth cycle for longer. Postpartum, oestrogen levels drop back to normal, causing many new mothers to experience hair loss for up to 6–12 weeks.

Hormones aren't the only cause though, with other contributing factors including excessive blood loss, lack of sleep, increased anxiety, high levels of stress and diet. It's currently thought about 50 per cent of us will notice a change.

To help us maintain a healthy head of hair we want to make sure that we're consuming a nutritious diet with adequate amounts of protein, iron and carbohydrates, along with healthy fats and a variety of vitamins and minerals too. Along with getting good sleep and finding ways to reduce anxiety, we can assist healthy hair growth by taking care of our scalp. Keeping the area washed, clean, hydrated and moisturised is important. For women with Afro-Caribbean hair, castor oil is often found to have a positive effect on stimulating cuticles.

Finally, if you feel your hair is being affected by postpartum shedding, be gentle with your hair styles. Try to avoid chemical products, the use of high heat and even limit brushing when possible. When brushing, starting at the bottom and working your way through the knots to the top is said to be a better way to comb then dragging from top to bottom, which may compound tangles, resulting in tougher brushing, exacerbating shedding.

Should I expect pre- and postnatal facial hair?

It's all starting to sound very glamorous isn't it! But, again, as with most of these points, any unusual facial hair is usually only temporary. It's all down to the hormonal changes taking place in our system. As such, women may find that hair begins to grow in unusual places during and after pregnancy. Often this begins towards the end of the second trimester. For many this resolves on its own by 6 months postpartum. If, however, you notice a marked increase after this time, it's worth a visit to your doctor to investigate whether there may be another cause and discuss treatment options.

Can my voice change after giving birth?

Some studies have found that a mother's voice drops by about two musical tones after pregnancy. Amazingly it's even been suggested that this is Nature's way of making sure a mother sounds more authoritative in her new role as a parent. Some women have reported noticing this change during pregnancy, although it's thought that the 'big drop' happens after delivery.

There has also been research to suggest that this change happens during our menstrual cycle as well, our pitch rising during ovulation each month. Our voices are then thought to decrease again following menopause.

Why this happens is unclear, although many are pointing the finger at hormone levels again. Not only could our hormones be directly affecting our vocal cords, but as pregnancy progresses, changes to our posture, reduction in lung capacity and the increased possibility of acid reflux all mean the sound of our voice can be impacted.

Will my breasts stretch and sag postpartum?

Okay, let's just tackle this question head on, no faffing around.

Will our breasts change in appearance postpartum? The short answer is, yes, for many of us there will be some change to our breasts after birth. I can't sugarcoat that bit; however, as you know, there is never a short answer when we're discussing pre- and postnatal health. There is so much more to know about our breasts during and after pregnancy. And if you're wondering whether your breasts will sag, not all women will experience the same. In fact, some women may even notice their breast size increase!

For many, however, pregnancy and breastfeeding can result in a drooping appearance of the breasts. Although contrary to what many believe, it's not actually that our breasts 'drop'; instead, during pregnancy the Cooper's ligaments that support a woman's breasts stretch due to the increase in size and weight of our breasts. This stretching of ligaments and skin may contribute to sagging breasts postpartum.

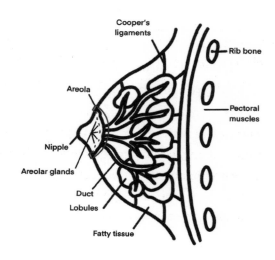

CAN EXERCISE HELP?

I have such a clear memory of someone telling me during pregnancy, 'Your breasts will never be the same.' I scoffed and rolled my eyes, putting this down to another fearmongering myth that women are subjected to; however, after a year of breastfeeding my first, I certainly noticed a change.

Exercise has always been my go-to treatment, for both my physical and mental wellbeing. But since breasts don't have muscle, we can't simply firm them up with exercise. There is, however, a network of connective fibrous tissue and surrounding muscle that can be worked and may help with appearance to a degree. Various chest exercises, as well as posture realignment and exercises such as swimming, can help to create support and strength around our chest.

WHAT ELSE CAN WE DO?

Getting adequate support is also crucial. Honestly, the simple act of being fitted for a bra in the correct size boosted my confidence after breastfeeding. A properly fitted bra adds support and reduces strain on the supportive tissue and muscle around our breasts. I remember being recommended a 'V'-shape cup as opposed to a balconette bra after breastfeeding my first son and I was happy to discover that my breasts instantly looked and felt more comfortable.

Should I expect vaginal dryness postpartum?

For something that is thought to affect around almost half of new mothers, it's surprising that this topic isn't spoken about more. There can be many contributing factors to vaginal dryness; however, as is often the case with pre- and postnatal changes, a substantial trigger is thought to be our hormones, particularly the role of oestrogen. Levels of oestrogen drop back to pre-pregnancy levels within 24 hours of giving birth; our body can dial these levels down even lower if we are breastfeeding, as oestrogen can interfere with milk production. Oestrogen is important to sexual arousal because it boosts the flow of blood to the genitals and increases vaginal lubrication.

This isn't, however, the only cause. Postnatal vaginal dryness can also be caused by a condition known as postpartum thyroiditis, which is the inflammation of the thyroid gland. This condition affects approximately 5 per cent of new mothers, and it can cause other symptoms such as difficulty sleeping, weight gain, depression, dry skin, fatigue, shakiness and heart palpitations.[37] If you feel you may be affected by this condition, it's worth raising with your GP who will be able to determine the underlying cause. Rest assured that, if affected, thyroid function typically returns to normal within 12–18 months for the vast majority of women.

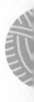

What are postpartum piles and are they common?

Postnatal haemorrhoids, also known as piles, are veins in the anus and lower rectum that have become swollen and engorged with blood. Many women experience them during pregnancy or postpartum for a variety of reasons including constipation, internal pressure or hormonal changes. They can range from irritating to quite painful, but there are no serious health risks associated with them. Some can go away with simple home treatments.

Piles appear in the rectal area and vary in size from about a pea to a grape. They are often caused as a result of stress on the perineum before, during and after birth. If you have any concerns speak with your GP, but to manage piles at home we can use simple measures such as cleaning the area gently but thoroughly, and eating lots of fibre to support soft and regular bowel movements. If needed we can apply ice to the area by wrapping an ice pack in a clean towel and applying for up to 10 minutes at a time, and using unscented and dye-free hygiene products like toilet roll or menstrual pads. If needed, using painkillers such as paracetamol is also considered safe during pregnancy.

After just a few weeks of diligent home care you should notice an improvement in your haemorrhoids; however, if symptoms persist aggressively or you experience any pain or rectal bleeding speak with your GP or midwife who will be able to explore further treatment options and investigate the leading cause.

❝ MOTHERHOOD CAN BE MESSY. IT'S A WONDERFUL, EMPOWERING, CHALLENGING, BEAUTIFUL BLESSING. ❞

What's the 'hot-mess' phase and how do I manage it?

I thought I'd round up this chapter with a phrase that a friend once told me that stuck in my head. On the surface, the situation we found ourselves in on that day didn't have much to do with motherhood.

I was being taught a dance routine by an old school friend and dance instructor, Bonnie Parsons (@bonnieparsons). We were collaborating on a 'feel-good' dance session for mums online and Bonnie told me, 'There's always a hot-mess phase in dancing. Which is where you've just learnt the routine. You go to perform it and forget a few steps, but rather than being embarrassed or shrinking into the background feeling like you've failed, style it out! Embrace the Beyoncé in you and work it!' Bonnie said the last bit with such flair that I instantly felt motivated.

We did the workshop and there were many times that I needed to embrace my 'hot-mess phase'. Still, I was elated and that natural euphoria stayed with me all day.

Later that afternoon, I needed to go to the supermarket, where I met a friend. After about an hour's shopping, I was at the till and the woman behind me tapped me on the shoulder and said, 'Excuse me, do you know you have a sticker on your forehead?' I felt my face and found a sticker of a cartoon dog right in the middle of my forehead. At first I laughed out loud. Then I realised that I'd had the sticker on my forehead for an hour in public. I felt embarrassed for about half a minute and then remembered Bonnie's words. I realised that I was living my hot-mess phase. I was right in the middle of mum mode and, you know what, I decided to style it out!

Motherhood can be messy. It's a wonderful, empowering, challenging, beautiful blessing and although at times things flow in synergy, sometimes we can find ourselves challenged. When the going gets tough, maybe we could all benefit from thinking a little more like Beyoncé and a little more like Bonnie, and embrace our hot-mess phase!

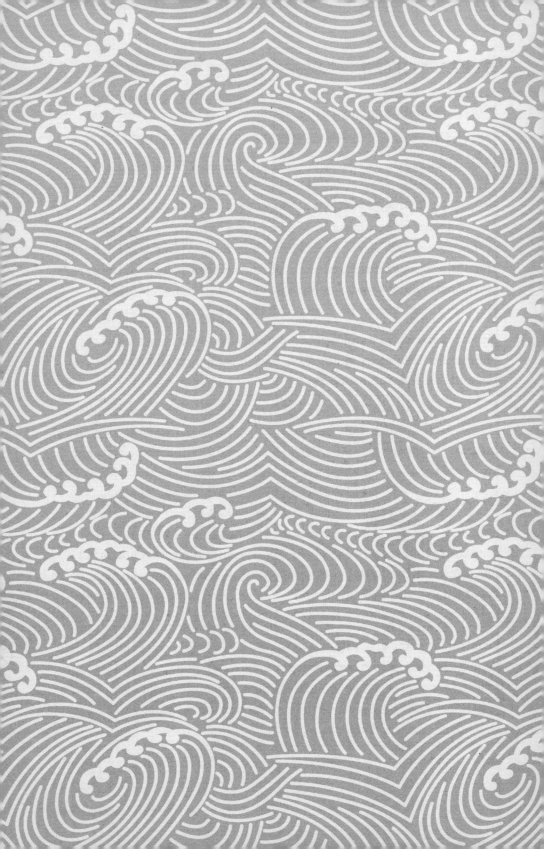

Before we wrap up

Before we wrap up, I wanted to write a little note, mother to mother.

Hopefully through this book you've picked up a few good pointers to help you lead a healthy pregnancy and recover postpartum.

When I started writing, I was determined to create something that not only spoke to women and gave them some support when they needed it, but that fuelled the fire inside each of us to confidently take our health into our own hands. I wanted to give every woman a little more clarity on how we can read the signals our body is giving us and then implement what's needed to help ourselves restore balance.

But they're not just words on the page. I would hate for you to end this book and feel uncertain of where to go next if you have other questions.

As I said right at the start, motherhood doesn't need to be a solo venture. They say it takes a village. Well, consider yourself my neighbour.

Because even though we're getting near the end, don't get ready to put me on the shelf just yet. I know that feeling of nearing the end of a read. I always feel a little nostalgic when that happens, especially when I've enjoyed it, which I hope you have, but motherhood is a community, with 24/7 access.

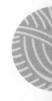

Seriously, we all know that when we're up in the middle of the night, there are millions of parents doing exactly the same thing! I used to think about that and feel less alone in those early hours of the morning.

In terms of what's next, first and foremost, thanks to technology, there are tons of ways to keep in touch. If you fancy it, you can always join the **StrongLikeMum** community online by heading over to stronglikemum. com or any other social media platform. I love to talk (if you hadn't realised already), so you'll always find me chatting about something related to pregnancy, postpartum or mum life, and I'll answer any questions I can (@shakira.akabusi).

Should something pop into your head suddenly, and you want quick answers or just need a reminder of some advice, you can flick back through these pages and find what you need. It might sound strange as you've just finished reading, but as each pregnancy and postnatal experience is different, you might find that you pick up new tips that feel more relevant every time.

We don't just need technology to keep in touch though. As mothers we're connected by something else as well.

Join the tribe

I started this book by travelling back millions of years to the days of Mitochondrial Eve and her companions, who were forming tribes and communities.

The human race may have branched out quite a bit since then, to countries and continents across the globe, but regardless of distance, we are united as mothers. Standing together and amplifying the power of women.

I've said countless times how unique every woman's pre- and postnatal journey is. That's the amazing thing about working in this industry. No one person's story is exactly the same as anyone else's. But even though no one will be experiencing exactly what you are, that doesn't mean we can't understand one another. We all still have common ground. Honestly, whatever you're experiencing or feeling, you are not alone.

The power of women, and more specifically mothers, never fails to amaze me.

I've been tested and pushed to my limits in motherhood, more than at any other time, both physically and mentally. But I've always found other people, most crucially mothers, to support me. And if you want it, you now have the exact same in me.

So, Mama, we're at the final page.

This isn't the end though. You're part of a sisterhood. You always have been, but hopefully now you feel it. I hear you.

Most of all, Mama, know this: your journey, your experience and your recovery matter.

This is just giving you that extra support.

Your health. In your hands. Alongside your tribe.

Shakira x

#StrongLikeMum

Acknowledgements

A huge thank you to Melanie Michael-Greer, my literary agent, for her endless patience, input and level-headed guidance through this mind-boggling journey of literature!

Thank you to the entire team at Little, Brown. With special thanks to my editor Tom Asker for supporting this book and allowing me to be so closely involved with the publishing process. Also to Rebecca Sheppard and Hannah Wood for their input with editing and the cover creation.

Thank you to Andrew Barron for his fantastic work on the internal design of the book.

To Sole De La Hoz (@drawnbysole) for her wonderful line drawings that bring the inside of the book to life.

To Attabeira (@attabeira_com) for creating artwork for the cover that speaks volumes and perfectly depicts the power of women and the essence of **StrongLikeMum**.

To my husband, for helping me complete this manuscript. Often by working late into the night himself so that I could nab a few hours during the day, and for being the most wonderful father to our children.

To my Mama and Papa, for inspiring me to believe I can have dreams and attempt to reach them. The idea of writing a book would have stayed purely that if I hadn't been encouraged to give things a go!

To my sister Ashanti, for her endless support in all that I do. For helping me to professionalise the initial pitch of this book and always having time when I needed to tease out some new web of ideas in my mind. And lots of love to all my siblings: Myron, Alannam and Sakhile.

Thank you to Helen Martin (@mother_of_copy), a fantastic friend and writer, for reading and re-reading this manuscript and sharing her golden nuggets of wisdom on how to work with words!

Thank you also to Vicky Sargent Designs (@vickysargent_designs) for sharing her knowledge and sparking the flames that laid the foundations for the design of this book.

To all my contributors, Katie Shore, Anna Mathur, Grace Hurry Pilates, Siobhan Miller, Catherine Rabess, Marie-Louise, Illiyin Morrison and to all the women I have worked with over the years who helped me learn everything I know today about the wonders of the female form.

Finally, to the entire **StrongLikeMum** community, online, in person and anyone who has bought or talked about this book. Everything I have learned has been down to the women I have worked with, trained and listened to. I will never be too old to stop learning and I am so grateful for everyone who has joined me on this journey.

Notes

1 Jane Gitschier, 'All about Mitochondrial Eve'. *PLoS Genetics*, May 2010. https://www.ncbi.nlm.nih.gov/pmc/articles/PMC2877732/

Rebecca L. Cann, Mark Stoneking and Allan C. Wilson, 'Mitochondrial DNA and human evolution'. *Nature* 325, 31–6 (1987). https://www.nature.com/articles/325031a0

2 https://www.psychologicalscience.org/publications/psychological_science

3 'Training Strategies for Your Female Clients After Abdominal and Pelvic Surgery'. Webinar hosted by MedFit Educational Foundation, presented by Jenice Mattek.

Jean-Philippe Gouin and Janice K. Kiecoult-Glaser, 'The impact of psychological stress on wound healing: Methods and mechanisms'. *Immunology and Allergy Clinics of North America* 31(1), 81–93 (2011). https://www.ncbi.nlm.nih.gov/pmc/articles/PMC3052954/

Ya-Ting Yang, Xiao-Li Wu and Wei Liu, 'Psychological stress enhances keloid development via stress hormone-induced abnormal cytokine profiles and inflammatory responses'. *Plastic and Aesthetic Research*, 7:34 (2020). https://parjournal.net/article/view/3553

4 Caitlin Thurber, Lara R. Dugas, Cara Ocobock, Bryce Carlson, John R. Speakman and Herman Pontzer, 'Extreme events reveal an alimentary limit on sustained maximal human energy expenditure'. *Science Advances* 5(6), (2019). https://www.science.org/doi/10.1126/sciadv.aaw0341

5 Laura Bailey, 'Childbirth an athletic event? Sports medicine used to diagnose injuries caused by deliveries'. *Michigan News*, 1 December 2015. https://news.umich.edu/childbirth-an-athletic-event-sports-medicine-used-to-diagnose-injuries-caused-by-deliveries/

6 Kelly R. Evenson et al, 'Guidelines for physical activity during pregnancy: Comparisons from around the world'. *American Journal of Lifestyle Medicine* 8(2): 102–21 (2014). https://www.ncbi.nlm.nih.gov/pmc/articles/PMC4206837/

7 Patrick J. O'Connor et al, 'Safety and efficacy of supervised strength training adopted in pregnancy'. *J Phys Act Health.* 8(3): 309–20 (2011). https://www.ncbi.nlm.nih.gov/pmc/articles/PMC4203346/

8 Roger Gadsby, Diana Ivanova, Emma Trevelyan, Jane L. Hutton and Sarah Johnson, 'Nausea and vomiting in pregnancy is not just "morning sickness": data from a prospective cohort study in the UK'. *British Journal of General Practice* 70 (697) (2020). https://bjgp.org/content/70/697/e534

9 J. Chang, Y. Zhang and Z. Lui, 'Impact of placental hormone withdrawal on postpartum depression'. *Zhonghua Fu Chan Ke Za Zhi* 30(6):342–4 (1995). https://pubmed.ncbi.nlm.nih.gov/7555367/

10 Healthline, 'What bodily changes can you expect during pregnancy?'. August 28, 2017. https://www.healthline.com/health/pregnancy/bodily-changes-during#hormonal-changes

11 Suchismita Chandran et al, 'Effects of serotonin on skeletal muscle growth'. *BMC Proceedings 2012*; 6 (Suppl 3): O3. https://www.ncbi.nlm.nih.gov/pmc/articles/PMC3394452/

12 Mustafa M. Husain, Diane Stegman and Kenneth Trevino, 'Pregnancy and delivery while receiving vagus nerve stimulation for the treatment of major depression: a case report'. *Annals of General Psychiatry* volume 4, Article number: 16 (2005). https://annals-general-psychiatry.biomedcentral.com/articles/10.1186/1744-859X-4-16

Allison Judkins, Rhaya L. Johnson, Samuel T. Murray, Steven Yellon and Christopher G. Wilson, 'Vagus nerve stimulation in pregnant rats and effects on inflammatory markers in the brainstem of neonates'. *Pediatric Research*, 83(2), 514–19 (2018). https://www.ncbi.nlm.nih.gov/pmc/articles/PMC5866172/

13 Royal College of Psychiatrists, *Post Natal Depression*. Royal College of Psychiatrists (2011). https://www.sth.nhs.uk/clientfiles/File/PostNatalDepression%5B1%5D.pdf

14 This was a survey carried out by Dove: https://www.dove.com/uk/baby/more-from-baby-dove/about-baby-dove/perfect-mum.html

15 Rachel Reiff Ellis, 'Does parent stress affect baby?' WebMD (2014). https://www.webmd.com/parenting/baby/features/stress-and-your-baby#1

Sara F. Waters, Tessa V. West and Wendy Berry Mendes, 'Stress contagion: Physiological covariation between mothers and infants'. *Psychological Science* 25(4), 934–42 (2014). https://www.ncbi.nlm.nih.gov/pmc/articles/PMC4073671/

S. F. Waters, H. R. Karnilowicz, T. V. West and W. B. Mendes, 'Keep it to yourself? Parent emotion suppression influences physiological linkage and interaction behavior'. *Journal of Family Psychology*, 34(7), 784–93 (2020). https://psycnet.apa.org/doiLanding?doi=10.1037%2Ffam0000664

Nicole R. Bush et al, 'Effects of Pre- and Post-natal Maternal Stress on Infant Temperament and Autonomic Nervous System Reactivity and Regulation In a Diverse, Low-Income Population'. *Development and Psychopathology* 29(5), 1553–71 (2017). https://www.ncbi.nlm.nih.gov/pmc/articles/PMC5726291/

16 Vera Sizensky, 'New survey: Moms are putting their health last'. healthywomen. org, March 27, 2015. https://www.healthywomen.org/content/article/new-survey-moms-are-putting-their-health-last

17 Moria Be'er, Dror Mandel, Alexander Yelak, Dana Lihi Gal, Laurence Mangel and Ronit Lubetzky, 'The effect of physical activity on human milk macronutrient content and its volume'. *Breastfeeding Medicine* 15(6), 357–61 (2020). https://pubmed.ncbi.nlm.nih.gov/32267727/

18 R. L. Gregory, J. P. Wallace, L. E. Gfell, J. Marks and B. A. King, 'Effect of exercise on milk immunoglobulin A'. *Medicine and Science in Sports and Exercise* 29(12):1596–1601 (1997). https://europepmc.org/article/med/9432092

19 J. P. Wallace and J. Rabin, 'The concentration of lactic acid in breast milk following maximal exercise'. *International Journal of Sports Medicine* 12(3):328–31 (1991). https://pubmed.ncbi.nlm.nih.gov/1889945/

20 Irene E. Hatsu, Dawn M. McDougald and Alex K. Anderson, 'Effect of infant feeding on maternal body composition'. *International Breastfeeding Journal* 3(2008). https://internationalbreastfeedingjournal.biomedcentral.com/articles/10.1186/1746-4358-3-18

Marian P. Jarlenski, Wendy L. Bennett, Sara N. Bleich, Colleen L. Barry and Elizabeth A. Stuart, 'Effects of breastfeeding on postpartum weight loss among U.S. women'. *Preventive Medicine* 69, 146–50 (2014). https://www.ncbi.nlm.nih.gov/pmc/articles/PMC4312189/

21 Carolyn A. Thomson and Kathy D. McCoy, 'The role of mom's microbes during pregnancy'. *The Scientist*, 1 Aug 2021. https://www.the-scientist.com/features/the-role-of-mom-s-microbes-during-pregnancy-69009

22 Iñaki Lete and José Allué, 'The effectiveness of ginger in the prevention of nausea and vomiting during pregnancy and chemotherapy'. *Integrative Medicine Insights* 11, 11–17 (2016). https://www.ncbi.nlm.nih.gov/pmc/articles/PMC4818021/

23 Giti Ozgoli, Marjan Goli and Masoumeh Simbar, 'Effects of ginger capsules on pregnancy, nausea and vomiting'. *Journal of Alternative and Complementary Medicine* 15(3):243–6 (2009). https://pubmed.ncbi.nlm.nih.gov/19250006/

24 Linghan Kuang and Yongmei Jiang, 'Effect of probiotic supplementation in pregnant women: a meta-analysis of randomised controlled trials'. *British Journal of Nutrition* 123(8):870–80 (2020). https://pubmed.ncbi.nlm.nih.gov/31856928/

Sara M. Edwards, Solveig A. Cunningham, Anne L. Dunlop and Elizabeth J. Corwin, 'The maternal gut biome during pregnancy'. *American Journal of Maternal/Child Nursing* 42(6) 310–17 (2017). https://www.ncbi.nlm.nih.gov/pmc/articles/PMC5648614/

Healthline, 'Should you take probiotics during pregnancy?' https://www.healthline.com/nutrition/probiotics-during-pregnancy#benefits

25 Elena A. Ponomarenko et al, 'The size of the human proteome: The width and depth'. *International Journal of Analytical Chemistry* 2016 (2016). https://www.ncbi.nlm.nih.gov/pmc/articles/PMC4889822/

26 NHS, 'Physical activity guidelines for adults aged 19 to 64'. https://www.nhs.uk/live-well/exercise/

27 Allanda, 'RCOG guidance on postnatal exercise'. 6 July 2011. https://www.allaboutincontinence.co.uk/blog/rcog-guidance-on-postnatal-exercise

28 James Owen, 'Humans were born to run, fossil study suggests'. *National Geographic*. 17 November 2007. https://www.nationalgeographic.com/science/article/humans-were-born-to-run-fossil-study-suggests

29 Amy Morin, 'As a psychotherapist, this is the biggest mistake I see people make when it comes to self-confidence'. 23 March 2019. https://www.inc.com/amy-morin/as-a-psychotherapist-this-is-biggest-mistake-i-see-people-make-when-it-comes-to-self-confidence.html

30 Daniel E. Lieberman, 'Is exercise really medicine? An evolutionary perspective'. American College of Sports Medicine (2015). https://scholar.harvard.edu/files/dlieberman/files/2015c.pdf

31 Sport England, 'New campaign to give women more confidence to exercise'. 2014. https://sportengland-production-files.s3.eu-west-2.amazonaws.com/s3fs-public/20150112-tgc-new-campaign-to-give-women-more-confidence-to-exercise.pdf

32 Avinash E. Thakare, Ranjeeta Mehrotra and Ayushi Singh, 'Effect of music tempo on exercise performance and heart rate among young adults'. *International Journal of Physiology, Pathophysiology and Pharmacology*. 9(2): 35–9 (2017). https://www.ncbi.nlm.nih.gov/pmc/articles/PMC5435671/

33 Friederike Mackensen, Wolfgang E. Paulus, Regina Max and Thomas Ness, 'Ocular changes during pregnancy'. D*eutsches Artzeblatt International* 111(33–34):567–76 (2014). https://www.ncbi.nlm.nih.gov/pmc/articles/PMC4165189/

34 NHS, 'Exercising in pregnancy'. https://www.nhs.uk/start4life/pregnancy/exercising-in-pregnancy/

35 Rebecca C. Thurston, James F. Luther, MA, Stephen R. Wisniewski, Heather Eng and Katherine L. Wisner, 'Prospective evaluation of hot flashes during pregnancy and postpartum'. *Fertility and Sterility* 100(6): 1667–72 (2013). https://www.ncbi.nlm.nih.gov/pmc/articles/PMC4167790/

36 Erin A. Wagner, Caroline J. Chantry, Kathryn G. Dewey and Laurie A. Nommsen-Rivers, 'Breastfeeding concerns at 3 and 7 days postpartum and feeding status at 2 months'. *Pediatrics.* 132(4): e865–e75 (2013). https://www.ncbi.nlm.nih.gov/pmc/articles/PMC3784292/

37 Sara Naji Rad and Linda Deluxe, 'Postpartum thyroiditis'. 20 June 2021. https://www.ncbi.nlm.nih.gov/books/NBK557646/

Index

Note: page numbers in **bold** refer to diagrams, page numbers in *italics* refer to information contained in tables.

postnatal checks 170–1, **170–1**
and postnatal posture pilates 196
and running 290–1
seated 170, **170**
standing 171, **171**
prams, buggy running 292–3
prebiotics 227–8
pregnancy
and abdominal muscles 49–52, **49, 51**
bleeding during 75, 213
and blood sugar balance 204–7, **205**
and blood volume 31–2, 68, 209, 211, 215
'bouncing back' from 16, 18
calorie requirements 218
and the core 25
energy requirements 25
exercises for 54–65
and the first trimester 68–75, 204–15
fitness 103
hormones 101–13
and nutrition 201–19
and the pelvis 29, 31–2
physicality of 45–65
running during 283
and the second trimester 75–85, 216–19
and skin tone 336
and sleep 174
and the third trimester 86–99, 218–19
and vision 334
water demands of 211
weight training during 77–8
'pregnancy glow' 32, 69
pregnancy tests 101–2
prenatal nutrition 201–19
press-ups
downward dog to modified press-up
258–9, **258–9**
elevated 82, **82**, 248–9, **248–9**
probiotics 216–17, 227–8
processed foods 184
progesterone 122–3
and the menstrual cycle 198, 199
as mood depressant 199
and night sweats 337
and pregnancy 102, 105–6
progress-monitoring 317–18
prolactin 117, 122, 135

protein 218, 225–6
Psychological Science (journal) 17
PTSD *see* post-traumatic stress disorder
ptyalism 335
purées 201

Rabess, Catherine 227–8
Rainbow Diet theory 207, 208
rapid eye movement (REM) sleep 175, 179
Rate of Perceived Exertion (RPE) 244–6,
245
RCOG *see* Royal College of Obstetrics and
Gynaecologists
recharging exercises 182–3
recovery 173–85
rectus abdominus 50–2, **51**
red blood cell production 69
red flags, and physical exercise 78–9, 245–6
relaxation 121, 130–1, 179–83, 323
jaw relaxation exercises 166–7, **166, 167**
standing foot relaxation exercise 166,
166
relaxin 107–11, 117, 197
reps 244
resistance band exercises 260–5
types of band 260
resistance band row 261, **261**
resistance training 282
rest 173–85, 322–3, 329
post-birth 156–7
reverse lunges 254, **254**
with dumbbell curl 273, **273**
with knee raise 81, **81**
root chakra (Muladhara) 33, 34
row
flat row 291, **291**
resistance band row 261, **261**
Royal College of Obstetrics and
Gynaecologists (RCOG) 211
RPE *see* Rate of Perceived Exertion
running 336
benefits of 280
buggy-running 292–3
during pregnancy 70, 283
and endurance 281–2
and the feet 287–9, **289**
and hydration 292

ACCESSIBLE, PRACTICAL ADVICE from
experts you can trust

The **Life Hacks** newsletter by **How To** is here to make your life easier and help you achieve the things that matter to you.

Each month we'll be sending you top tips and life hacks on topics ranging from cookery to personal finance and everything in between. Also keep your eyes peeled for giveaways, book offers and much more.

SIGN UP TO THE NEWSLETTER TODAY
www.howto.co.uk/landing-page/how-to-newsletter/

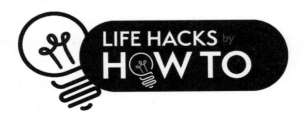